A PRACTICAL GUIDE TO THE SELF-MANAGEMENT OF LOWER BACK PAIN

A Holistic Approach to Health and Fitness

JAMES TANG

authorHOUSE®

AuthorHouse™ UK
1663 Liberty Drive
Bloomington, IN 47403 USA
www.authorhouse.co.uk
Phone: 0800.197.4150

© 2018 James Tang. All rights reserved.

No part of this book may be reproduced, stored in a retrieval system, or transmitted by any means without the written permission of the author.

Published by AuthorHouse 08/10/2018

ISBN: 978-1-5462-9542-6 (sc)
ISBN: 978-1-5462-9543-3 (hc)
ISBN: 978-1-5462-9541-9 (e)

Library of Congress Control Number: 2018908856

Print information available on the last page.

Any people depicted in stock imagery provided by Getty Images are models, and such images are being used for illustrative purposes only.
Certain stock imagery © Getty Images.

This book is printed on acid-free paper.

Because of the dynamic nature of the Internet, any web addresses or links contained in this book may have changed since publication and may no longer be valid. The views expressed in this work are solely those of the author and do not necessarily reflect the views of the publisher, and the publisher hereby disclaims any responsibility for them.

CONTENTS

Preface xi
Acknowledgements xv
Introduction xvii
    What Is Lower Back Pain? xviii
    Prevalence xviii

Chapter 1 - Causes of Lower Back Pain 1
    1.1 Common Causes of Lower Back Pain 1
    1.2 Classification of Lower Back Pain 3
    1.3 Typical Symptoms of Musculoskeletal Lower Back Pain 3

Chapter 2 - Physiology of Muscle Contraction 5
    2.1 Introduction 5
    2.2 Types of Muscles 5
    2.3 Type of Fibres in Skeletal Muscles 6
    2.4 Motor Unit Recruitment and the All-or-None Law 9
    2.5 The Sliding Filament Theory 10
    2.6 Length-Tension Relationships of Muscles 11
    2.7 Muscle Dysfunction 12
    2.8 The Human Movement System (HMS) 13

Chapter 3 - Musculoskeletal Lower Back Pain 14
    3.1 Common Causes of Musculoskeletal Lower Back Pain 14
    3.2 Muscle Imbalances 16
        3.2.1 Common Causes of Muscle Imbalances 17
    3.3 Core Dysfunction 19
        3.3.1 Benefits of Core Stability 20

- 3.3.2 Anatomy of the Core 20
  - 3.3.2.1 The Deep Muscles of the Spine 22
  - 3.3.2.2 The Middle Muscle Layer (The Inner Unit) 22
  - 3.3.2.3 The Outer Muscle Layer (Outer Unit, Global Muscles) 24
- 3.3.3 Integrated Core Function 26
- 3.3.4 Common Causes of Core Dysfunction 26
- 3.4 Functional Roles of Muscle Contractions 27
- 3.5 Reciprocal Inhibition 29
- 3.6 Synergistic Dominance 30

Chapter 4 - Self-Management of Lower Back Pain 32
- 4.1.1 General Advice on Self-Management of Lower Back Pain 32
- 4.1.2 Simple Exercises for Alleviation of Acute Lower Back Pain 35
- 4.1.3 Identification of the Cause of Your Lower Back Problems 38
- 4.1.4 Corrective Exercises for Lower Back Pain 41
- 4.2 Inhibitory Phase 42
  - 4.2.1 Background 42
  - 4.2.2 Myofascial Pain Syndrome 42
  - 4.2.3 Adhesions of Fascia 42
    - 4.2.3.1 Fascia 42
    - 4.2.3.2 Myofascia 43
    - 4.2.3.3 Treatment of Adhesion Using Self Myofascial Release (SMR) 44
  - 4.2.4 Trigger Points 44
    - 4.2.4.1 Symptoms of Trigger Points 47
    - 4.2.4.2 Prevalence of Trigger Points 48
    - 4.2.4.3 Characteristics of Trigger Points 48
    - 4.2.4.4 Causes of Trigger Points 50
    - 4.2.4.5 Types of Trigger Points 51
    - 4.2.4.6 Treatment of Trigger Points Using (SMR) 52
    - 4.2.4.7 Physiology of SMR 53
    - 4.2.4.8 How Long Does It Take to Get Relief from Trigger Points? 53
  - 4.2.5 The Relationship between Fibromyalgia (FM) and Trigger Points 55

4.2.6 Practical Advice on Self Myofascial Release 56
    4.2.6.1 The Ten-Second Press Test 56
    4.2.6.3 SMR of Deep Spinal Muscles 59
    4.2.6.4 SMR of Erector Spinae 60
    4.2.6.5 SMR of the Quadratus Lumborum (QL) 62
    4.2.6.6 SMR of Gluteal Muscles 66
4.2.7 Cupping Therapy 71
4.3 Lengthening Phase 74
  4.3.1 Introduction to Flexibility 74
  4.3.2 Practical Advice on Stretches 77
    4.3.2.1 Hamstring Stretch 78
    4.3.2.2 Hip Flexor Stretch 80
    4.3.2.3 Adductor Stretch 82
    4.3.2.4 Tensor Fasciae Latae (TFL) and Iliotibial Band
          (IT Band) Stretch 84
    4.3.2.5 Piriformis Stretch 86
    4.3.2.6 Quadratus Lumborum (QL) Stretch 88
    4.3.2.7 Erector Spinae Stretch 89
    4.3.2.8 Rectus Femoris Stretch 91
4.4 Activation Phase 93
  4.4.1 Introduction to Activation 93
  4.4.2 Practical Advice on Activation 94
    4.4.2.1 Activation of Gluteal Muscles 94
    4.4.2.2 Activation of the Quadratus Lumborum (QL) 99
    4.4.2.3 Activation of the Transversus Abdominis (TvA) .. 100
  4.4.3 Core-Strengthening Exercises 101
4.5 Integrated Dynamic Movements 108
  4.5.1 Core Stability 108

Chapter 5 - Obesity and Back Pain 116
5.1 Introduction to Obesity and Back Pain 116
5.2 Metabolism and Macronutrients 118
  5.2.1 Carbohydrates 120
  5.2.2 Fats 122
  5.2.3 Protein 123
    5.2.3.1 Protein Supplements 123

5.3.1 Creatine Phosphate, or Phosphocreatine, System
(CP System) 125
5.3.2 Lactate System 125
5.3.3 Aerobic System 126
5.3.4 How Does Diet Contribute to Weight Loss? 127
5.3.5 How Does Stress Affect Your Weight? 128
5.3.6 Diet and Exercise 128
5.4 Exercises for Weight Loss: Cardiovascular Exercises 130
   5.4.1 Warm-Up 131
   5.4.2 Cardio Training Zones 132
5.5 Exercises for Weight Loss: High-Intensity Interval
   Training (HIIT) 137
   5.5.1 Types of Interval Training 143
   5.5.2 Cool-Down 146
5.6 Exercises for Weight Loss: A Beginner's Guide to the Principle of
   Resistance Training 147
   5.6.1 Dynamic Stretches 148
   5.6.2 Repetitions (Reps) 149
   5.6.3 Pros and Cons of Various Resistance Exercises
   (Machines or Free Weights) 153
   5.6.4 The Concept of "Balance Training" 154
   5.6.5 Effects of Resistance Training 155
   5.6.6 Sample Full-Body Resistance Training 157
   5.6.7 Types of Muscle Contraction 159
   5.6.8 Advanced Resistance Training Techniques 160
   5.6.9 How Body Type Influences the Response to Training
   and Weight Loss 167
      5.6.9.1 Ectomorph 167
      5.6.9.2 Mesomorph 168
      5.6.9.3 Endomorph 168

Chapter 6 - Postural Dysfunction 171
6.1 Introduction to Posture 171
6.2 Common Postural Deviations 175
   6.2.1 Hyperlordosis 175
   6.2.2 Hyperkyphosis 178

    6.2.3 Scoliosis 182
    6.2.4 Sway Back Posture.. 183
    6.2.5 Military Posture 184
    6.2.6 Slumped Posture 184
    6.2.7 Flat-Back Posture.. 184
    6.2.8 Cumulative Injury Cycle (Diagram 6.2.8)............................ 184
  6.3 Corrective Exercises for Hyperlordosis 186
  6.4 Corrective Exercises for Hyperkyphosis 190

Chapter 7 - Flat Feet and Lower Back Pain 199

Chapter 8 - Sacroiliac Joint Dysfunction and Lower Back Pain 204
  8.1 Functional Anatomy of the Sacroiliac Joints (SI joints) 204
  8.2 Causes of SI Joint Pain 205
  8.3 Symptoms and Diagnosis of SIJ Problems 206
  8.4 Corrective Exercises for Lower Back Pain Resulting from SI Joint
      Dysfunction 207

Chapter 9 - The Best Way to Sleep for Lower Back Pain Sufferers..... 209
  9.1 Ideal Sleep Positions to Ease Your Lower Back Pain 209
  9.2 Pillow Strategies 211
  9.3 Mattresses for Lower Back Pain 212

Further Reading 213
Endnotes 223

PREFACE

Having worked as a dentist for a couple of decades with poor posture, I have been suffering from back pain for over twenty years. In fact, my interest in lower back pain began when I injured my back some twenty years ago when lowering a piece of luggage. I was astounded by the pain, which was so intense and debilitating that I struggled to get out of bed on the following morning. I simply could not turn my body. The experience was truly frightening, and it took a whole week to get better. But most worryingly, my back became so vulnerable that even minor tasks, such as bending down to pick something up from the floor, could trigger a severe episode of intense back pain which would last for weeks.

The problem was exacerbated by the fact that no one was able to offer me any constructive and consistent advice. The information that I obtained was piecemeal, inconsistent, and at times contradictory. For instance, my doctor told me to rest or to take painkillers, while although my physiotherapist did eradicate my acute symptoms and recommended certain exercises, he never explained the rationale behind these activities. I was told by a personal trainer at my gym to strengthen my back muscles and core. I followed the advice of my fellow gym-goers by foam rolling my back, but I did not really know what I was doing. I was completely bewildered by the conflicting advice and simply could not understand why my back problems would recur even though I was complying with the various instructions. I am sure that this frustration is ubiquitous.

I was so fed up that I subsequently decided to take control of my predicament by learning to manage my own back problems. I have since become a personal trainer, sports massage therapist, and NASM corrective exercise specialist. Inspired by my success in reversing my recurrent lower back pain, and fuelled by a vibrant enthusiasm to share my knowledge with those who suffer from these stubborn musculoskeletal problems, I began to passionately research how to holistically manage musculoskeletal pain and learnt a wealth of information. I have lectured on postural dysfunction and musculoskeletal conditions for many years, helping my fellow colleagues in the dental profession to improve their postures to prevent musculoskeletal pain. I have written numerous articles for various dental magazines including the British Dental Journal (BDJ), BDJ Team, BDJ in Practice, The Dentist, Dentistry, Private Dentistry and The Probe. I have contributed articles to the newsletters of the Dentists' Provident Society and the Medical Defence Union of Scotland, and to a webinar hosted by KaVo Dental.

I am aware that there are many books available on the subjects of lower back pain, core-stability exercises, flexibility training, trigger point management, and cardiovascular and resistance training etc., but there is really no such literature on the holistic approach to the self-management of lower back pain; a practical guide that integrates all the different modalities in one logical and systematic programme, firstly by recognising the possible cause of the predicament, and secondly by effectively managing it to prevent recurrence. I have reviewed many articles on the relationships between poor posture and prolonged static posture on the causation of lower back pain, but none of them mention how such risk factors contribute to back problems, nor do they offer any practical advice on the effective management of these conditions.

You may not be suffering from any lower back pain at present but prevention is always better than cure and I hope you will find the content of this book beneficial.

Purpose and limitations of this book

We need to be aware that everyone's lower back pain condition is unique; the cause of such problems is not the same as different muscle groups are implicated. There is therefore no single solution for these ailments.

This is not intended to be a reference or academic textbook and I will endeavour to make this guide as practical and relevant as possible. Furthermore, it is not the intention of this book to offer any diagnoses or treatments. Although trigger points (section 4.2.4) are implicated in the majority of cases of muscular pain, there may be underlying conditions which must be addressed by the medical profession. You are therefore advised to consult your doctor, physiotherapist, or other relevant professional if you suffer from any form of back pain. You can then use this self-help guide to assist you to understand the treatment protocol and rationale behind the rectification strategies being offered.

The information in this book is provided purely from the perspective of an exercise professional, sports massage therapist, and musculoskeletal pain sufferer. I am not medically qualified and the contents of this book are for general information only and should not be considered as a medical opinion.

This book will help you to understand the common causes and symptoms of lower back pain and the general principles of self-management that relate to these conditions. The management strategies offered are generalized and are not specific to you. Therefore, the book should not be used to self-diagnose or self-treat any health, medical or physical condition. You can appreciate that unless a thorough examination and postural analysis have been carried out, it is impossible to establish a definitive diagnosis or to offer a bespoke rectification plan. Please therefore consult your healthcare or exercise professional before embarking on the corrective activities recommended in this book.

For example, you should not go ahead and activate underactive tissue until you know which groups of muscles are underactive. Similarly, you should not stretch your tight tissues unless you know what is actually causing the tightness. Let me give you a pertinent example of why professional advice is important: if your hamstrings are tight, this could be due to an anterior tilting of your pelvis, probably as a result of hyperlordosis (section 6.2.1), pulling on the hamstring thus making it tight. Stretching this muscle without consciously rectifying your anterior pelvic tilt or your hyperlordotic posture may worsen your pelvic misalignment because a stretched hamstring will simply allow the pelvis to tilt forward even further. In this situation, you should first have your anterior pelvic tilt corrected by consciously correcting your hyperlordosis and by strengthening your glutes and abdominal core (section 4.4.2), before stretching out your hamstrings.

To complicate things further, your anterior pelvic tilt could be caused by problems further down your kinetic chain. For example, flat feet (chapter 7) may be causing internal rotation of your knees and anterior tilting of your pelvis. In this case, you first need to have your flat feet problems attended to by a podiatrist.

In a nutshell, there is no one-size-fits-all concept for dealing with your lower back problems. Professional advice must be sought in the first instance if you have any musculoskeletal pain.

Only a limited number of corrective exercises and stretches have been selected as examples, and numerous alternatives are available. It is clearly not possible to list every single type of exercise in this book and to go through their detailed execution. You are advised to engage an exercise professional who is experienced in corrective exercises for postural dysfunction as they will be able to design a bespoke rectification protocol for you. Furthermore, it is important to follow the correct execution and progression of these exercises to ensure effectiveness and to avoid injury.

ACKNOWLEDGEMENTS

I feel honoured and privileged to have been able to produce this book. As you can imagine, like most books, it has taken many painstaking hours to put together, and finally it is done.

My gratitude also extends to my family and medical friends who gave me inspiration and supported me as I embarked on my journey to write a book on lower back pain. It is my fervent hope that my past experience of pain will help other sufferers.

I must thank my ex-boss, an eminent dentist for whom I have the greatest respect (although he wishes to remain anonymous, he has spent a lot of time and effort reviewing this book and has provided me with pertinent and invaluable suggestions). My gratitude also goes to Dr Peter Savage, my daughters Jenny and Carey, and Mr Paul Rooney for reviewing the content of the book. Jenny also generously took the majority of the photographs for me while I demonstrated the various corrective exercises. Finally, thanks to David Lloyd Newcastle for allowing me to use its gym and studio for filming.

For regular updates, please visit my website or contact me on
www.healthaddiction.co.uk
For regular tips on health and fitness, please follow me on Instagram – **james.tang90**
Please subscribe to my YouTube Channel – **'James Tang Fitness'**, where I will regularly upload the corrective exercises for postural dysfunction as mentioned in the book.

INTRODUCTION

"What could be better than transforming a person's life?" – This motto inspired me to write this book which advocates a holistic approach to health and fitness.

Paraphrasing John F. Kennedy, the thirty-fifth president of the United States, I invite you to ask not what your back can do for you; rather, ask what you can do for your back. He said this because he had a lifelong struggle with chronic back pain. Back pain is common, but if you ignore it, it can become chronic and can adversely affect your entire life.

The problem is that we often choose to pay no notice to our symptoms because we are so preoccupied with work, family, and other pressing matters; our backs are the last thing we worry about.

We spend a long time at work in front of our computers, sitting on cheap non-ergonomic chairs, hunching over with our eyes staring at the screen. We neglect to move about even when the little aches come along to remind us that it's time to stretch and relax a little.

At the beginning, your back may just be a little sore. Then it feels stiff, and the movement of your torso becomes more restricted. Then, you start feeling your back muscles going nuts and seizing up, causing you to bend over like an old man, unable to move. Soon it may even become chronic, and you may think you have to live with it for the rest of your life and constantly take medication like JFK.

I do not want this to happen to you. That's why I wrote this practical guide, in which I share my experience to employ corrective exercises to reverse the damage of bad posture and lower back pain and prevent it from recurring.

What Is Lower Back Pain?

Lower back pain is defined as **pain, muscle tension or stiffness localized between the areas covered by the 12th rib and gluteal fold**. Sometimes, lower back pain is accompanied by pain going down the leg, a condition known as **sciatica** (section 4.3.2.5). Back pain can actually occur in any area of the back, where there is a stack of twenty-six vertebrae connected by ligaments, muscles and shock-absorbing intervertebral discs. All structures that make up the spine may contribute to your back pain, but it is more common to have pain in the lower back, as this supports most of the body's weight.

Prevalence

If you have back pain, you are in the majority of the general population. Estimates vary, but approximately 60 to 80 per cent of us will get at least mild back pain at some time in our lives, and this is a significant cause of lost work and productivity. Back pain causes high levels of anxiety and discomfort, and it has been linked to depression. There is a great deal of conflicting advice, and patients are often left confused, in pain, and compelled to seek help.

Unlike arthritis where the problem is clear to both patients and surgeons as the pathology can be identified on radiographs (x-rays), back pain is a problem for sufferers because they often cannot get clear and consistent advice on its causes or the rectification protocols. This is an issue for medical professionals because they cannot identify any definite pathology, establish the exact source of the pain or offer any real cure. This is also a problem for the macroeconomy as lower back pain is one of the most common reasons for lost work, healthcare usage, and the payment of sickness benefits.

CHAPTER 1
Causes of Lower Back Pain

1.1 Common Causes of Lower Back Pain

The back is a complex framework, and the lumbar spine, or low back, is a remarkably well-engineered structure of interconnecting bones, joints, nerves, ligaments, and muscles all working in synchrony to provide support, strength, and flexibility, thus allowing your centre of gravity to be maintained over a constantly changing base of support during functional movements. However, this complex structure also makes the lower back vulnerable and susceptible to injury and pain.

It is quite difficult to make an accurate diagnosis as to the exact nature of back pain; even with the use of the latest imaging and other types of test, doctors are often unable to pinpoint the precise cause. On the other hand, it is possible that imaging tests such as magnetic resonance imaging (MRI) will show problems in the spine of a patient who has no back pain.

Back pain is therefore a symptom rather than a disease on its own. Most back pain is musculoskeletal in origin, although pain that arises from other organs may be felt in the back. Many intra-abdominal disorders, such as appendicitis, aneurysms, kidney diseases, bladder infections, pelvic infections, cancer, and ovarian disorders can cause pain that is referred to the back, but these rarely present as back pain alone. There are nearly always some associated gastrointestinal, urinary, or gynaecological symptoms. For example, a previous dental patient of the author had experienced lower back pain for months and had rightly sought medical advice. Unfortunately, his general practitioner dismissed it as pain which was being caused by muscle overexertion and he simply told him to rest. As expected, the condition persisted and worsened, and months later, his back condition was diagnosed as being caused by pancreatic cancer.

Finding the optimal treatment for lower back pain very much depends on obtaining a correct diagnosis that identifies the underlying cause of the symptoms. Although it is not the intention of this book to offer any diagnoses or treatments, the general consensus is that if you suffer from any form of lower back problems, especially when it is persistent or exhibits the following symptoms, you must seek immediate medical advice.

- History of cancer with recent weight loss not due to lifestyle changes, such as diet and exercise
- Fever and chills
- Pain from your lower back being referred elsewhere such as down your buttocks and legs
- Severe trauma
- Significant leg weakness
- Loss of bladder and bowel control
- Severe, continuous abdominal pain and back pain.

Additionally, if you experience pain after a major trauma, such as a car accident, or if your lower back pain is so severe that it interferes with your daily activities, mobility, or sleep, or if there are any other troubling symptoms, you should seek medical attention immediately.

This book will concentrate only on the most common cause of lower back pain—**musculoskeletal** pain—which is generally caused by **muscle dysfunction** (section 2.7) when muscles are not contracting properly or applying the right amount of force during contraction, but where there is no specific pathology such as nerve compression or herniation of discs.

1.2 Classification of Lower Back Pain

Besides classifying back pain according to the location of discomfort—upper, middle, or lower back—it can usually be classified according to duration and recurrence:

Acute back pain refers to pain that has been felt for less than six weeks. Acute symptoms tend to come on suddenly, usually in response to an event such as a slip, awkward twist or injury. They generally last for a few days to a few weeks, and often resolve on their own, even without treatment. However, recurrence is common. The initial pain can be so severe that you may not be able to turn or get out of bed with ease, but please be assured that while your current pain is intense and your functional mobility is restricted, you can usually recover in a few days with the correct treatment, activities, and advice (sections 4.1.1 and 4.1.2). But for avoidance of recurrence, you need to manage your lower back condition with the holistic approach advocated in chapter 4.

- Subacute back pain persists for between six weeks and three months.
- Chronic back pain persists for more than three months.
- Frequent episodes are classed as recurrent back pain.

1.3 Typical Symptoms of Musculoskeletal Lower Back Pain

Back pain has a marked effect on sufferers, as well as on society, due to its prevalence and economic consequences. But, if you are unfortunate enough to suffer from lower back pain, how can you tell if your condition is due to a serious spinal injury (which luckily accounts for less than 1 per cent of all back pain[1]) or another systemic illnesses, such as a tumour? Generally speaking, if the pain persists for more than six weeks, is constantly intense, gets worse, or is accompanied by any of the symptoms mentioned above in section 1.1, you should definitely seek medical attention.

Those who have suffered from musculoskeletal back pain may recall these familiar symptoms:

- Generally, the pain varies with time and physical activity. The back is usually stiff in the morning; after you have been moving about, it improves. Conversely, for non-musculoskeletal causes of lower back pain, the discomfort tends to be constant; rest or exercises do not relieve it, and you may not be able to find any position of comfort.
- The pain does not affect general health, such as causing fever or sudden and unexplained weight loss.

Musculoskeletal lower back pain usually presents in patients between twenty to fifty-five years of age. Patients who present before the age of twenty are more likely to have a serious disease or a structural problem, such as spondylolisthesis, a condition in which one's vertebra slides forward over the bone below it that most often occurs in the lower spine. Patients who develop new or different back pain after the age of fifty-five are more likely to have a serious diseases, in particular from cancer that has spread to the spine (spinal metastasis), or osteoporosis.

The majority of sufferers (including the author) tend to have recurrent symptoms because this type of pain is strongly associated with trigger points (section 4.2.4). Research by Drs Janet Travell and David Simons, authors of *The Trigger Point Manual*, has shown that trigger points are the primary cause of pain in at least 75 per cent of the cases and are a factor in nearly every painful condition. Without intervention, trigger points do not disappear; they simply turn latent and can be reactivated with the slightest stress or strain. This explains why although acute episodes generally settle down, even without treatment, after a week or so, the pain may not fully disappear and recurrence is common. It is therefore imperative that you do not simply concentrate on the elimination of pain, even though this may appear to be your most urgent need, but that you also manage the condition effectively (chapter 4).

CHAPTER 2
Physiology of Muscle Contraction

2.1 Introduction

In order to understand how muscles become dysfunctional and how trigger points are formed (section 4.2.4), you need to understand the basic physiology of muscles function; you can then start to help them heal using corrective exercises (chapter 4).

2.2 Types of Muscles

There are three types of muscle in our bodies: smooth, cardiac and skeletal.

Smooth Muscles

Smooth muscles are involuntary due to our inability to control their movements. They are found in the walls of hollow organs such as the stomach, oesophagus and bronchi, and in the walls of blood vessels.

Cardiac Muscle (Heart Muscle)

This type of muscle is found solely in the walls of the heart. It is under the control of our autonomic nervous system, which regulates a variety of body process that take place without conscious effort. But even without a nervous input, contractions due to the pacemaker cells can take place. The cardiac muscle is highly resistant to fatigue due to the presence of a large number of mitochondria (structures in cells where respiration happens) and myoglobin (a globular protein that serves to bind and deliver oxygen), and a good blood supply allowing continuous aerobic metabolism.

Skeletal Muscles

Skeletal muscles attach to bones and contract to facilitate movement of the skeleton. They are also known as striated muscles because of the stripy appearance resulting from bands of actin and myosin forming the sarcomere (the basic functional unit within muscle cells) within the muscle cells, the myofibrils.

These muscles are voluntary, meaning we have direct control over them through our nervous system. They consist of 70 per cent water, 23 per cent protein (actin, myosin, and collagen) and 7 per cent minerals.

2.3 Type of Fibres in Skeletal Muscles

Within skeletal muscles, there are three types of fibre.

Slow-Twitch (Type 1) Fibres (The Local Muscular System—for Stabilization)

Stabilizer muscles

Stabilizer muscles are not confined to the spine and are not movement specific. They provide stability to allow movement of a joint. An example of this is the rotator cuff muscles of the shoulder that provide dynamic stabilization for the humeral head (the head of the humerus – the long bone in the upper arm located between the elbow joint and the shoulder) in the glenoid fossa (a shallow depression in the scapula, or shoulder blade, where the humeral head articulates).

Postural Muscles

Examples of postural muscles include the core musculatures, such as the transversus abdominis, multifidus, internal oblique, diaphragm, and the pelvic floor muscles (section 3.3.2.2). These muscles are primarily composed of type 1 aerobic fibres that are used for endurance-type activities. They are loaded with myoglobin (which gives them their red appearance) and mitochondria. They therefore use oxygen and fat as their main fuel source for contraction (section 5.3.3). The myoglobin is able to increase the rate of oxygen diffusion so red slow-twitch fibres are able to contract for longer periods. These fibres do not generate as much force as type 2 fibres but are more resistant to fatigue. For this reason, the muscles containing primarily type 1 fibres are often postural muscles and have an antigravity role and are heavily involved in the maintenance of posture. In addition, athletes such as marathon runners have a high number of this type of fibre, partly through genetics and partly through training.

Most problems with muscle shortening occur in postural muscles because, with the correct posture, these muscles are fairly inactive and only respond to disruptions in the balance to maintain an upright position. Therefore, when you move away from ideal alignment, postural muscle tone is increased (chapter 6).

Fast-Twitch (Type 2) Fibres (A and B)—The Global Muscular Systems (Movement Systems)

Fast-twitch fibres consist of more superficial musculatures that are larger and are associated with movements of the torso and limbs. They primarily consist of two main types of fast-contracting muscle fibres: type 2a and type 2b. Both are able to produce fast, strong muscle contractions, but are quick to fatigue.

Fast-twitch type 2a fibres have a fast contraction speed and can use aerobic, or oxygen-dependant (section 5.3.3), energy sources, as well as anaerobic, or oxygen-independent (sections 5.3.1 and 5.3.2), energy sources. These are known as "white fibres", as they are low in myoglobin and less reliant on oxygen supplied by the blood for energy, and therefore they fatigue faster than slow-twitch fibres.

Fast-twitch type 2a fibres are suited to speed, strength, and power activities, such as moderately heavy weight training (eight to twelve reps, section 5.6.2) and fast running events, such as the four hundred metres. Fast-twitch and slow-twitch fibres cannot be converted into each other. However, type 2a fibres (intermediate fibres) can adapt in different ways depending on the type of training performed. In response to endurance training, they will adopt the characteristics of slow-twitch fibres; and in response to resistance training, they can turn from type 2a fibres into type 2b fibres.

Type 2b fibres are often known as fast glycolytic fibres. They are white in colour owing to the low level of myoglobin and a relative lack of mitochondria. Muscles composed primarily of this type of fibre are called global muscles. Type 2b fibres produce ATP (adenosine triphosphate, section 5.3) at a slow rate by anaerobic metabolism and they break it down very quickly. This results in short, fast bursts of power, and rapid fatigue.

Like type 2a fibres, the fast-twitch type 2b fibres are also suited to speed, strength, and power activities. Heavy weight training (one to three reps), power lifting, and one-hundred-metre sprints are examples of activities that predominantly require 2b fibres.

Movement is the main function of global muscles; they are more superficial, tend to span several joints, and are composed primarily of type 2b fibres. A tight postural muscle often results in inhibition (section 3.5) of these global muscles, whose function becomes weakened as a result. A typical example of this is tight hip flexors inhibiting the function of the glutes. When trying to correct a musculoskeletal imbalance, you should encourage lengthening of an overactive muscle prior to attempting to strengthen a weak elongated muscle.

We are genetically programmed to have a certain percentage of each muscle fibre type. It is thought that the average person is born with around 60 per cent fast-twitch fibres and 40 per cent slow-twitch fibres; those who are born with a higher amount of fast-twitch fibres are more suited to power activities, while those with a higher percentage of slow-twitch fibres are more suited to endurance activities, such as marathons and triathlons.

Furthermore, the proportion of slow- and fast-twitch fibres in each muscle is determined by its role. The muscles of the neck and back have a key role in the maintenance of posture and so have a high proportion of slow-twitch fibres, which are slow to fatigue. The muscles of the shoulders and arms are often used to generate force, and they have a higher proportion of fast-twitch fibres. Although there is a distinction between postural and global muscles, many muscles can exhibit characteristics of both and contain a mixture of type 1 and type 2 fibres. For instance, leg muscles (quadriceps, hamstrings, and the calf muscles) often have high numbers of both fast- and slow-twitch fibres, since they must both continually support the body and play a role in movement. The hamstring group of muscles, for instance, has a postural role and is notoriously prone to shortening.

Generally speaking, muscles that have a stabilizing role (postural) have a tendency to shorten when stressed. Other muscles that play a more active or motive role (global) have a tendency to lengthen and become inhibited (e.g., the gluteus maximus).

2.4 Motor Unit Recruitment and the All-or-None Law

A motor unit consists of a single motor neuron (a nerve fibre that effects muscle contraction) and all the muscle fibres it innervates (supplies). When a nerve impulse travels down a neuron (nerve cell), all the muscle fibres within that motor unit are activated. So the motor unit either activates all of its fibres or none at all. This is known as "the all-or-none law."

The number and size of motor units in specific areas of the body depends upon their functional roles. For example, postural muscles have fewer motor units supplying more fibres, and those muscles that are involved in more intricate movements, such as those of the hands, have more motor units supplying fewer fibres.

<u>Effect of Exercise on Motor Unit Recruitment</u>

One of the long-term adaptations to resistance training (section 5.6.5) is the enhancement of neuromuscular connections by recruitment of more motor units. This adaptation will enable the muscle to generate more strength during contractions.

2.5 The Sliding Filament Theory

The most basic unit of a muscle is the muscle cell, which is known as the myofibril.

Muscle contraction begins when a nervous impulse arrives at the neuromuscular junction—a place in the body where the axons of motor nerves meet the muscle, allowing them to transmit messages from the brain that cause the muscle to contract and relax. This impulse causes a release of a neurotransmitter called acetylcholine, which in turn causes the depolarization of the motor end plate. This leads to the release of Calcium (Ca+) from the sarcoplasmic reticulum—a system of membrane-bound tubules that surrounds muscle fibrils, releasing calcium ions during contraction and absorbing them during relaxation.

Within each myofibril are strands of myofilaments called actin and myosin. They are arranged in a series of compartments called sarcomeres that run the length of the myofibril (diagram 2.5). The actin is anchored to the end of the sarcomere, and the myosin sits within the middle of the sarcomere. These filaments slide in and out between each other to cause muscle contractions. Millions of sarcomeres have to contract in your muscles to cause even the smallest movement. In the presence of high concentrations of Ca+, the Ca+ binds to troponin, changing its shape and so moving tropomyosin from the active site of the actin. The myosin filaments can now attach to the actin, forming a cross-bridge.

The breakdown of ATP releases energy (section 5.3), enabling the myosin heads to attach themselves to the actin filament and rotate, pulling the actin filaments inward towards the middle to generate tension. This occurs along the entire length of every myofibril in the muscle.

The myosin detaches from the actin, and the bridge is broken when an ATP molecule binds to the myosin head. When the ATP is then broken down, the myosin head can again attach to an actin binding site further along the actin filament and repeat the "power stroke".

This process of muscular contraction can last for as long as there is adequate ATP and Ca+ stores. Once the impulse stops, the Ca+ is pumped back to the sarcoplasmic reticulum and the actin returns to its resting position, causing the muscle to lengthen and relax. It is worth noting that an increased release of calcium ions is postulated to be an essential part of trigger point formation (section 4.2.4). A trigger point exists when overstimulated sarcomeres become unable to change out of their contracted state.

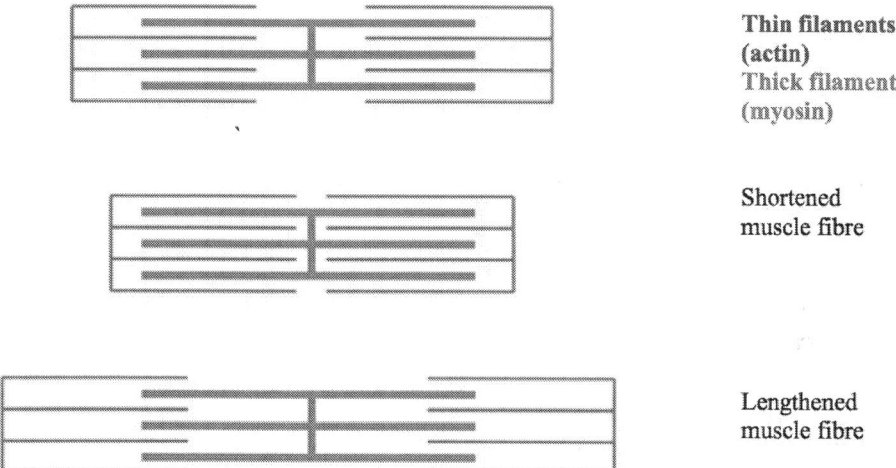

Diagram 2.5 Sliding filament theory of muscle contraction

2.6 Length-Tension Relationships of Muscles

The length-tension relationship in a muscle is the relationship between the length of a muscle fibre and the force that it produces at that length. When a muscle fibre is stretched to the point of minimal overlap of contractile protein actin and myosin, the contraction force will be weakened. Similarly, when a muscle is shortened, the contractile force will also be weakened.

Therefore, muscles can become weak because they are stretched or are too tight. Muscles are more prone to injury, fatigue and damage when they are weak.

As we will be able to see in subsequent chapters, spending an excessive amount of time in a seated position will not only affect the length-tension relationships of muscles that are attached to the lumbo-pelvic-hip complex, it can ultimately lead to reduction in core muscle activation (section 3.3) owing to a lack of neural stimulation. Therefore, even relatively light loads placed upon these muscles exceed their ability to cope, as they have been "inactive" for so long.

2.7 Muscle Dysfunction

Muscle dysfunction essentially means abnormality in muscle function, either not contracting properly or not applying the right amount of force during contraction, but there is no pathology.

Muscles are dysfunctional and weakened if they are stretched for a prolonged period of time. Likewise, muscles are dysfunctional and weak if they are contracted for a prolonged period of time, causing muscle tightness. Furthermore, when these muscles are tight, there is a reduction in blood flow, making it difficult for them to accomplish their basic physiological functions, including the removal of waste that would naturally be carried away in the blood. Additionally, the muscles are deprived of oxygen, which is essential for tissues to remain healthy. A lack of oxygenated blood being delivered to a muscle will exacerbate its dysfunction, result in increased muscle fatigue, and impede the muscle repair process and the ability to recover from exercise. All these factors can greatly increase the chances of injury.

Essentially, muscle adaptation means that shortened muscles can, over time, become structurally short and mechanically incapable of lengthening to an appropriate level. Overstretched muscles can become structurally long and incapable of shortening to an appropriate level.

When muscles are incapable of firing correctly, compensation occurs, and this will alter joint motion from its normal path, resulting in the cumulative injury cycle (section 6.2.8).

2.8 The Human Movement System (HMS)

The human movement system (HMS)[2] is a complex, well-orchestrated system of interrelated and interdependent myofascial, neuromuscular, and articular components. The functional integration of each system allows for optimal neuromuscular efficiency during functional activities. Optimal alignment and functioning of all components results in an ideal length-tension relationship and neuromuscular control. The HMS consists of the muscular system, the skeletal system, and the nervous system. Throughout your body, rarely does a single muscle work without other muscles contributing. This is because the everyday functioning of the body is an integrated and multidimensional system. For example, during functional movements, the body must maintain the alignment of its centre of gravity over a constantly changing base of support. If a change in alignment occurs at one joint, changes in alignment at another joint must occur in order to compensate. Consequently, impairment in one system or a component of each system can lead to compensation and adaptation in other systems, initiating the cumulative injury cycle (section 6.2.8), the repair process that our body goes through to heal an injury, causing decreased performance and musculoskeletal pain. Furthermore, when an articular structure is out of alignment, the joint surfaces will be subjected to abnormal stress, and this may lead to osteoarthritis over time.

CHAPTER 3
Musculoskeletal Lower Back Pain

3.1 Common Causes of Musculoskeletal Lower Back Pain

Most back pain is simply a mechanical disturbance of the musculoskeletal structures of function of the back but without specific pathology. This type of lower back pain is far more common than those with pathological causes (section 1.1). The increasing degree of automation has led to greater amounts of sedentary time and time spent in static postures. In the past, the main reason for lower back pain was lifting heavy loads with a poor posture. Nowadays, more and more people are suffering from lower back pain due to long occupational sedentary time, and a static sitting posture. Let us now examine the most common causes of this type of back pain.

Wear and tear: Due to daily activities or direct trauma to a particular area, especially with sudden or jerking movements that place too much stress on the lower back. Other examples of activities that can cause wear and tear include accidents, falls, fractures, sprains, dislocations, and direct blows to the muscle.

Sports injuries (especially in sports that involve twisting or significant forces of impact): Please note that with any long-standing or chronic pain, there will be compensations and adaptations in a range of muscles locally and even remotely from the pain area.

Improper lifting techniques: This can include lifting heavy objects or twisting the spine while lifting.

- **Poor sleeping habits** (chapter 9): Such as sleeping with an improper posture or habitually curling up in bed for a prolonged period (this posture is particularly common when you sleep in a cold room without adequate heating).
- **Emotional stresses:** We all respond to stress in different ways. Some people react to stress in their minds, but others hold stress in their body, and it can affect their neck and back. The cause of neck and back pain as a result of stress or anxiety is mostly secondary, meaning that the stress is not literally causing the pain, but is causing behaviours that lead to this pain. When you are stressed, you automatically tense up in the shoulder and neck region. As a result, you extend the cervical (neck) portion of the spinal column forward. If you feel depressed, you hold your head down and become too relaxed in this area. These positions can cause muscle imbalances, ultimately leading to musculoskeletal neck pain or even spinal disc problems. You may also begin to tense your back muscles, which can trigger or exacerbate lower back pain. In fact, stress and lower back pain can create a vicious cycle; if you have back pain and you begin to worry about it; this causes stress, and your back muscles begin to tense. Tense muscles exacerbate your back pain, and you worry more, which makes your back worse, and so on. Furthermore, stress may change your behaviours and posture, including the way you sit and whether you slouch etc. Changes in posture can cause tension in the muscles, which can ultimately lead to back pain (chapter 6). Furthermore, stress may change your activity levels, which can play a direct role in the causation of lower back pain (see below).
- **Lack of activity and a sedentary lifestyle:** Exercises are essential because intervertebral discs receive no blood supply and they derive their nutrition by diffusion caused by compression and decompression. The longer you sit or stand without moving or changing your posture, the worse it is for your discs. Furthermore, regular exercises, both strengthening and stretching, maintain the

mobility and flexibility of all the joints, thus helping to reduce the prevalence of musculoskeletal disorders (section 4.3.1).
- **Smoking:**[3] Nicotine may affect the manner in which the brain processes sensory stimuli and the central perception of pain. But how does smoking increase the chances of you suffering from lower back pain? We know that the more demand an activity or load places on the spine, the more likely it may become injured, resulting in pain. This is why those who are obese (chapter 5) and those with heavy occupational workloads tend to be associated with lower back pain. However, we also need to consider how well the body can recover from minor damage, and one of the keys to healing is ensuring that an injured area of the body has an adequate blood supply to provide the resources and nutrients for healing. Smoking may damage tissue in the lower back and elsewhere in the body by slowing down circulation and reducing the flow of nutrients to joints and muscles.

Besides the abovementioned factors, by far the most common causes of musculoskeletal lower back pain are muscle imbalances and core dysfunction.

Let us take a look at these in more detail.

3.2 Muscle Imbalances

Movements occur through a coordinated contraction of muscles around a joint. Muscles are generally set up with one group needed to perform a given activity, such as flexing your leg (hamstrings) and another group used for the opposing action, such as extending your leg (quadriceps).

Almost every bodily movement has a possible opposite movement (known as the agonist/antagonist relationship, section 3.4). Muscular pairs which accomplish these opposing movements can work front to back or side to side (left and right) throughout the body.

Imbalances occur when one set of specific task musculature is overdeveloped while the opposing muscles are underdeveloped, resulting in some muscles being shortened or tight and others being lengthened or stretched. In both cases, the muscles are dysfunctional and weakened (section 2.6).

Although muscle dysfunction is one of the major causes of musculoskeletal pain, the concept of muscle imbalance is not well recognized. The advice you receive for the management of this type of pain can therefore often be contradictory; it not only fails to bring you long-term pain relief, but it can often aggravate your back condition. For example, the author was instructed by his personal trainer to strengthen his back in order to eradicate his back pain. Whilst this may be true in general, if your back problem is caused by your overtightened lower back muscles, as in the case of hyperlordosis (section 6.2.1), strengthening them will simply worsen the situation. It must therefore be reiterated that it is of the utmost importance that you seek professional advice to establish the cause of your back pain before you embark on any corrective exercises.

3.2.1 Common Causes of Muscle Imbalances

<u>Poor Posture</u>

Postural dysfunction is one of the most common causes of muscle imbalances. Optimal posture must be maintained at all times—not only when holding static positions, but also during functional activities. Long-term poor static postural habits (section 6.2) alter the length-tension relationship of muscles (section 2.6) that are attached to the lumbo-pelvic-hip complex. In these circumstances, the muscles become dysfunctional (section 2.7) and will not be able to generate proper force for efficient movement.

Unfortunately, postural dysfunction is common in our modern lifestyles of sitting hunched over computers all day, driving, and then spending evenings on the couch, watching television. This means that certain muscles, often postural muscles (e.g., the hip flexors), are chronically tight, and others are often weak—typically global muscles composed of predominantly type 2 fibres (e.g., the gluteus maximus). A lot of people are acutely aware of this issue but the majority do not really know how to address their postural problems. You need to be aware of what is the ideal posture to adopt (Section 6.1) and then consciously use it in your daily routines. Correcting your incorrect posture will inevitably feel awkward at the beginning because you are so used to sitting and standing in a certain way. But it is essential that you be aware of your postural deviations and get this corrected consciously.

Obesity

Obesity affects both adults and children. We are well informed that obesity is inextricably related to the development of certain fatal diseases, such as coronary heart disease, diabetes, and high blood pressure, but we may not be aware that obesity can also contribute to, or worsen lower back pain. This is because abdominal obesity shifts the centre of gravity forward, causing an increase in the natural lordotic lumbar curve and anterior tilting of the pelvis. This leads to imbalances of muscles that are attached to the lumbo-pelvic-hip complex (section 6.2.1). Such postural deviations also lead to faulty loading patterns, which increase the strain on the spine and the associated joints. Losing weight therefore means less stress on joints, tendons, and muscles. Furthermore, being overweight is often associated with being sedentary, which can limit the strength and flexibility of the back (section 4.3.1), making it more susceptible to injury.

Prolonged Sitting and a Sedentary Lifestyle

In order to grasp the reason why prolonged sitting is detrimental, it is important to understand how muscles adapt to the positions that we put them in. The longer we hold a certain position, the more tissue adaptation occurs, leading to muscle imbalances (section 3.2). Muscles can therefore become adaptively shortened or lengthened, depending on the position. This is because our bodies are not designed to maintain the same body position or engage in repetitive movement patterns hour after hour, day after day. But, unfortunately, we often cannot avoid prolonged static postures either at work or at home. Human beings are four-limbed animals, and like our cousins, we are designed to move around and hunt for food; if we put a gorilla in a chair all day, it may get a bad back too!

Other causes of muscle imbalance due to prolonged sitting include a poor sitting posture. The majority of us do not sit upright with a neutral spine. We may even cross our legs or slouch while we sit, resulting in a posterior tilting of the pelvis leading to even greater disc and muscle imbalances.

<u>Incorrect Resistance Training Strategies</u>

Muscle imbalances are also often seen in the gym when people focus on one muscle group more than another; when the muscles on one side are stronger than those on the other, you have muscle imbalance. The stronger muscles pull that part of your body out of position and your whole body ends up making adjustments to compensate, ultimately leading to postural dysfunction. A good example of this is when people overemphasize the training of their pectorals (chest muscles), deltoids (shoulders) and biceps. Tight pectorals can predispose them to hyperkyphosis (section 6.2.2), typically associated with round shoulders, forward head posture, and internal rotation of the shoulder joint, leading to a decrease in subacromial space and impingement of the supraspinatus and infraspinatus tendons of the rotator cuff muscles, predisposing people to shoulder pain.

Please refer to section 5.6 for a beginner's guide to the principles of resistance training.

3.3 Core Dysfunction

Another common cause of musculoskeletal lower back pain is core dysfunction. The core is a system of stabilization. Although the core muscles are primarily in the centre of your body, the core affects your entire body.

When you stand, your postural muscles contract to regulate your posture and maintain your balance. But if you sit on a stable surface for a prolonged period of time, especially when you sit on a chair with a backrest, the core muscles are no longer required to maintain your balance or to stabilize the spine. Over time, these core musculatures become weakened and dysfunctional. Furthermore, the majority of those who go to the gym commonly use exercises to develop strength only in the superficial muscles composed primarily of type 2 fibres (section 2.3), neglecting the flexibility (section 4.3.1) and strength of the core (section 4.4.3).

The core is often misunderstood as being only the rectus abdominis, commonly known as the "six-pack". However, the core simply means "the ability of your trunk to support the effort and forces from your arms and legs during functional activities, thus allowing your muscles and joints to perform in their safest, strongest, and most effective positions". It is important because any movement that uses the whole body requires a strong core to stabilize the spine and to transfer power between the upper and lower halves, through the pelvis.

3.3.1 Benefits of Core Stability

The benefits of core stability are as follows:

- **Improved performance**: Whether you enjoy an occasional gym session or whether you are an elite athlete, core stability should be an integral part of your training. Working on your core can vastly improve balance and torsion (twisting) strength, and can significantly enhance your performance in activities like racket sports, dancing, and swimming.

- **Injury prevention**: Bracing your core at all times during functional activities is essential to prevent injury to the lower back area. When you activate your core, the rest of the muscles in the area, such as the hamstrings, gluteal muscles, and other abdominal and back muscles, all work more efficiently together.

Rehabilitation from injury: Core stability is an essential component of any rehabilitation programme for lower back pain sufferers, as it provides deep stability to the superficial global muscles that initiate movements.

3.3.2 Anatomy of the Core

There are two distinct yet interdependent systems that enable our bodies to distribute forces efficiently. These systems include the local muscular system, also known as the stabilization system, and the global muscular system, the movement system (section 2.3).

In order to fully understand the function of the core, we firstly need to examine the anatomy of the stabilizing ligaments and muscles of the spine.

- Anterior longitudinal ligaments connect each vertebral body together and run anteriorly along the spine, preventing excessive spinal extension (backward bending of the torso).
- Posterior longitudinal ligaments run along the posterior aspect of the spine and underneath the spinous processes, helping to prevent excessive spinal flexion.
- Interspinous ligaments connect each spinous process to the one immediately above or below, together with the posterior longitudinal ligament, preventing excess spinal flexion (forward bending of the torso).
- Intertransverse ligaments connect each transverse process to the one immediately above or below. These ligaments run on either side of the spine and help to prevent excess lateral flexion (sideways bending of the torso).

These passive structures are much weaker than muscles and can therefore withstand only a small amount of force. The muscular system is therefore primarily responsible for maintaining core stability and posture.

The Muscles of the Spine

The muscles of the lower back help stabilize, rotate, flex, and extend the spinal column, a bony system comprising twenty-four vertebrae that gives the body structure and houses the spinal cord. Put simply, there are three layers of muscles: deep, middle, and outer. It is the coordinated contraction of these muscles that determines the level of safe and effective core function.

3.3.2.1 The Deep Muscles of the Spine

The movements of the spine and limbs can be divided into two categories: physiological and accessory. Examples of gross physiological movements include flexion and extension of the torso, running, jumping, and lifting. Accessory movements occur alongside physiological movements but take place within each vertebral segment. To control these intricate accessory motions, there are a number of smaller, deeper muscles in close proximity to the spine that connect one vertebral segment to another:

- Intertransversarii attach between the transverse processes of the vertebrae. They help to bring about lateral flexion and control smaller movements between vertebrae. They also aid in stabilizing the spine.

- Interspinales attach between the spinous processes of the vertebrae. They are located on either side of the interspinous ligament. They assist in bringing about spinal extension and control the smaller movements between vertebrae. Like the intertransversarii, the interspinales play a significant role in spinal stabilization. But unlike the intertransversarii, the interspinales help stabilize the spine while it is moving, in a process known as dynamic stabilization.

- Rotators attach from the spinous process of one vertebra to the transverse process of the vertebra immediately below. They help to bring about rotation between spinal segments and help to control the smaller movements between vertebrae.

3.3.2.2 The Middle Muscle Layer (The Inner Unit)

This local muscular system is the prime component of the core musculature; it comprises muscles that are predominantly involved in support and stabilization of the spine and which do not provide gross physiological movements. This layer includes the following:

- **Diaphragm:** This is a dome-shaped muscle separating the thoracic and abdominal cavities. It contracts downward and helps create intra-abdominal pressure to stabilize the spine.

- **Pelvic floor:** The pelvic floor is a group of muscles at the base of the pelvis that hold the organs and provide a sling running from back to front, from the bottom tip of the spine (the tail bone) to the front of the pelvis. It contracts simultaneously with the transversus abdominis to form the bottom of the cylinder of muscles.

- **Transversus abdominis (TvA,** section 4.4.2.3)**:** This is the deepest of all the abdominal muscles, and it forms a corset around the trunk region, lying deep to the rectus abdominis (six-pack). It functions by drawing the waist in, compressing the abdominal contents, and increasing intra-abdominal pressure to stabilize the spine. The TvA appears to be the key muscle of the core. Richardson et al (1999)[4] discovered that in individuals with no back pain, the TvA fired 30 milliseconds prior to shoulder movements and 110 milliseconds prior to leg movements. The key role of the TvA is to provide core stability for functional activities of the limbs.

- **Multifidus:** The multifidus starts at the base of the spine at the sacrum and extends up to the second vertebra in the neck. It is a series of smaller muscles that connect the spinous processes to the transverse processes of the spine. They are the largest and most medial of the lumbar back muscles. One important physiological function of this muscle is to take pressure off the vertebral discs and to create padding between vertebrae so the body's weight can be evenly distributed. It helps to provide rotation and extension of the spine and to hold the lumbar segments in an extended position. Both the multifidus and the TvA link with the thoracolumbar fascia—a large area of connective tissue, roughly diamond shaped, which comprises the thoracic and lumbar parts of the deep fascia enclosing the intrinsic back muscles, to provide a deep muscle corset that protects the back from injury.

These middle-layer muscles co-contract to raise the intra-abdominal pressure, creating a non-compressible cylinder where the spine is stabilized and forming the working foundation from which the limbs can function satisfactorily and safely. It is like an inflated balloon compressing against the spine and stabilizing it. This intra-abdominal "balloon" (diagram

3.3.2.2) has the diaphragm at the top, the pelvic floor muscles at the bottom, and the transversus abdominis (TvA) forming the surrounding walls; the multifidus muscles are positioned posteriorly. Faulty inner unit recruitment increases the likelihood of lower back dysfunction.

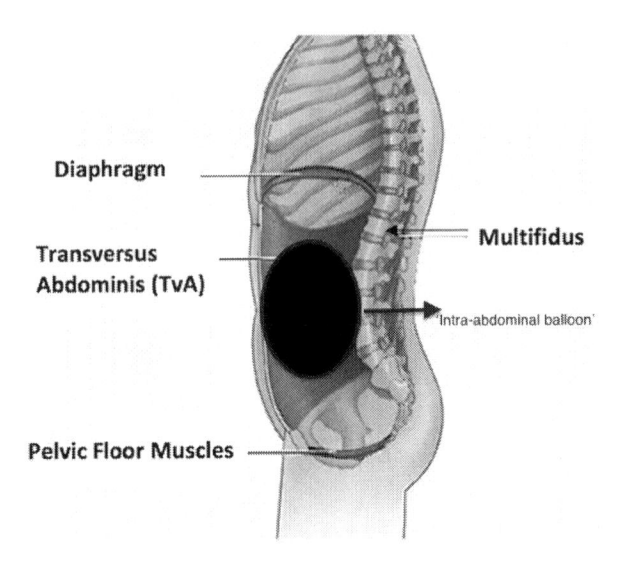

Diagram 3.3.2.2—Muscles of the core

When all these muscles contract together, they keep the spine in its most stable position, and aid in preventing injury. They should contract prior to any functional movements of the limbs, and they function in keeping the torso rigid and stable during all functional movements.

3.3.2.3 The Outer Muscle Layer (Outer Unit, Global Muscles)

This system is predominantly responsible for movement of the trunk and extremities. It primarily consists of large superficial musculature, such as the rectus abdominis, latissimus dorsi and external obliques.

The movements of these muscles are recruited by the nervous system as groups known as **muscle synergies**. Muscles do not work in isolation because it is more effective to allow muscles and joints to operate as an integral unit. For example, when you extend your shoulder (i.e., move your arm back), the latissimus dorsi, teres major and posterior deltoid all work together as an integral unit to perform the action.

Just a bit of extra information that you may be interested in: our bodies consist of four muscle synergies – the lateral subsystem, the deep longitudinal subsystem, the posterior oblique subsystem, and the anterior oblique subsystem (table 3.1).[5]

Subsystems	Components	Role
Lateral-	Gluteus medius, tensor fascia latae, adductors and contralateral (opposite side) quadratus lumborum (QL)	Frontal plane stability and pelvic-femoral stability during single-leg movements, such as in gait, lunges, or stair-climbing
Deep Longitudinal	Erector spinae, thoracolumbar fascia, sacrotuberous ligament, and bicep femoris (of the hamstrings)	Stabilize the body from the ground up. It provides force transmission longitudinally from the foot and ankle to the trunk and back down. It controls ground reaction forces during gait.
Posterior Oblique	Gluteus maximus, latissimus dorsi, and thoracolumbar fascia	Works synergistically with the deep longitudinal subsystem distributing transverse plane forces created through rotational activities.
Anterior Oblique	Internal oblique, external oblique, adductor, and hip external rotators	Like the posterior oblique subsystem, this system also functions in a transverse plane, but from the anterior portion of the body. When we walk, our pelvis must rotate in the transverse plane in order to create a swinging motion for the legs. This rotation comes in part from the posterior oblique posteriorly and the anterior oblique subsystem anteriorly. This system is also important in stabilizing the lumbo-pelvic-hip complex.

Table 3.1: The Four Global Muscle Subsystems

It is important to be aware that we simultaneously use all four of these subsystems during functional activities, epitomizing the fact that the human movement system is an integrated system (section 2.8). This explains why impairment in one system, such as that due to muscle dysfunction, can lead to adaption and compensation by another system (section 3.6), resulting in the initiation of the cumulative injury cycle (section 6.2.8) and musculoskeletal problems, such as neck, shoulder, and lower back pain.

Furthermore, the effective operation of the four subsystems of the outer unit is dependent upon the proper functioning of the inner unit for the stability that is necessary to create an effective force generation platform.

As previously mentioned in section 2.3, the outer unit muscles are primarily responsible for gross physiological bodily movements, such as flexion, extension, and rotation of the spine. They mainly comprise type 2a and 2b fibres, which are strong but quick to fatigue. They are therefore not designed for postural activities, which is the primary role of the deeper core muscles composed primarily type 1 fibres.

3.3.3 Integrated Core Function

If the muscles of the core do not contract in the right order, or the deeper core muscles lack strength, this can lead to an over-reliance on large, global muscles (such as the rectus abdominis) lying more superficially to stabilize the trunk which can create muscle spasms of the inner unit, as they have been inactivated or dysfunctional. Dysfunction of the core is therefore a common cause of lower back pain.

3.3.4 Common Causes of Core Dysfunction

Besides prolonged sitting on stable surfaces, core dysfunction is often present in those who incorrectly use sit-ups as a core-training exercise.

When you perform sit-ups, stabilizing and mobilizing muscles are trained in roles opposite those they were designed for. The rectus abdominis (commonly known as the "six-pack"), a predominantly type 2 fast-twitch muscle that is normally active in strength and explosive tasks, is mainly responsible for this action. They are being used to perform the required action repetitively in an endurance-type capacity, resulting in fast-twitch muscles taking on the role of slow-twitch muscles. This often weakens the deeper core muscles, such as the TvA. The rectus abdominis tries to perform both stabilizing and mobilizing roles, thus "switching off" the deeper core muscles, leading to back pain due to dysfunction of the core musculatures.

Core stability exercises (section 4.5.1) are designed to train our core muscles, which should ideally work together in a coordinated manner.

3.4 Functional Roles of Muscle Contractions

Before we discover how muscle imbalances and core dysfunction actually lead to lower back pain, let us first analyse the four functional roles of muscle contractions.

To create specific movements of the joints, muscles exert a force and pull on the bones. We already know that throughout the body, rarely does one group of muscles work without other muscles contributing, because movement occurs through a coordinated contraction of a number of muscles around a joint.

Let us take the example of a bicep curl. When your biceps (biceps brachii) contracts, your arm flexes. In this case, the prime mover is the biceps, which contracts to cause the desired action.

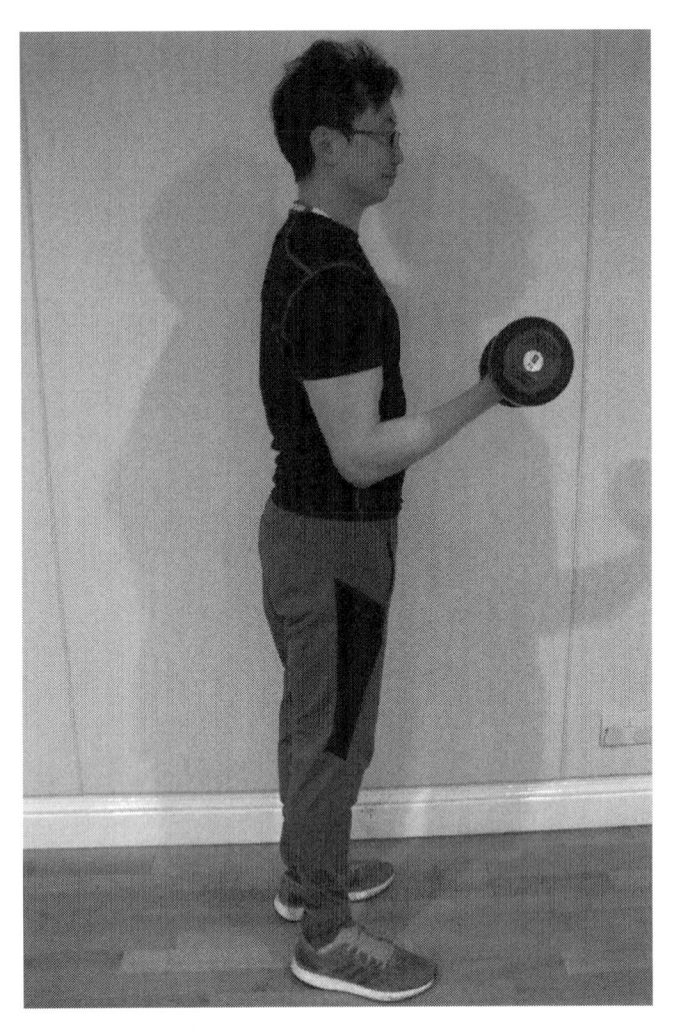

Diagram 3.4: Bicep Curls

- **Agonist:** .The agonist is the prime mover. This muscle contracts and causes a desired action. For instance, when you contract your biceps, it creates flexion of your arm. It is important to be aware that a muscle can only be referred to as an agonist in relation to a movement. It is inappropriate to label any one muscle as an agonist unless we are describing its role in a movement. So saying "the biceps brachii is an agonist" in isolation is incorrect, because the biceps brachii is an antagonist when we extend our arm when the triceps becomes the agonist in this movement.

- **Antagonist:** The antagonist is the muscle opposing the agonist that relaxes during movement. This is usually a muscle that is located on the opposite side of the joint from the agonist. The triceps, an extensor of the elbow joint, is the antagonist for elbow flexion.
- **Synergist:** A synergist contracts to assist the movement of the prime mover. The most important aspect of understanding how muscles function to produce a joint movement is **synergy**. Synergy means that two or more elements work together to produce a result that is greater than any of those components could achieve alone, so that the whole result is greater than the sum of the individual effects of the component involved. In our example of the bicep curl, the synergists are the brachialis and brachioradialis. (We will soon learn about how synergist muscles of the back contribute to lower back pain.)
- **Fixator:** Also known as a stabilizer or neutralizer. These contract to stabilize the part of the body that remains fixed. Fixators basically help movement by opposing unwanted movement or by helping to stabilize the joint. For example, deltoids (shoulder muscles) dynamically stabilize the shoulder when the arm moves.

3.5 Reciprocal Inhibition

Reciprocal inhibition is a neuromuscular reflex that inhibits opposing muscles during movement. For example, if you contract your elbow flexors (biceps brachii), then your elbow extensors (triceps) are inhibited. Reciprocal inhibition therefore describes the process of muscles on one side of a joint relaxing to allow contraction on the other side of that joint.

Through reciprocal inhibition, when one muscle shortens, its antagonist will always lengthen. If you have a muscle that is constantly shortened in a given context, the antagonist will be lengthened within that context. This is how a tight muscle can inhibit the function of its counterpart.

3.6 Synergistic Dominance

We already know that muscles work in groups because movement occurs through the coordinated contraction of a number of muscles around a joint.

To put it simply, if the agonist, or prime mover, does not contract properly, then the brain will look for alternative solutions to create the same movement, resulting in the synergist or the helper muscles taking over the role of the prime mover. This phenomenon is known as synergistic dominance. This is a temporary solution to ensure that the correct movement occurs, but synergists are not designed to be the agonist, and they are less efficient. Over time, this can lead to dysfunctional movement patterns and formation of trigger points in these muscles due to overexertion, which can result in injury and pain (section 6.2.8).

<u>A Typical Example of Synergistic Dominance due to Prolonged Sitting</u>

Our bodies are very efficient and will adapt to any stresses that we place upon them. When these stresses are balanced, the body will remain in balance. Dysfunctions can start with muscle imbalances; for instance, when you sit, your hip is in a flexed position and your hip flexor muscles, the **iliopsoas** (section 4.3.2.2), become tight; and the glutes (section 42.6.6), the antagonists of hip flexion, become inhibited through reciprocal inhibition.

The glutes are primarily responsible for hip extension (moving your legs backwards), hip stabilization, and eccentric deceleration of hip flexion (i.e., opposition of the force of the hip flexors). They are required to work when you run or walk. If your glutes are switched off, weak, or are not functioning properly, other helper muscles take over when you walk, run and climb stairs. Synergists, such as the hamstrings (section 4.3.2.1), quadratus lumborum (QL, section 4.2.6.5), erector spinae (section 4.2.6.4), and piriformis (section 4.3.2.5) substitute and become overactive. The formation of trigger points (section 4.2.4) within these synergist muscles as a result of their overactivity is one of the most common causes of lower back pain.

Of course, this is just a simplistic overview of what can happen with prolonged sitting. If you slouch when you sit, you can end up with a posterior pelvic tilt with lengthened back muscles and tight abdominal muscles, with both of these groups of muscles being weakened (section 2.7). Conversely, if you sit with excessive lumbar extension, you end up with an anterior pelvic tilt with shortened and tight back muscles (erector spinae) and stretched core and abdominal muscles (rectus abdominis and transversus abdominis) (section 6.2.1). If you sit with your torso twisted, with a wallet placed in your back pocket on one side whilst you sit, or with your legs crossed, you may suffer from lateral pelvic tilt and stress to your sacroiliac joints (chapter 8). The list goes on and on and it would be impossible to go through every single scenario. The objective of this section is to give you an overview of the effect of prolonged sitting, both at work and at home, and the effect of poor sitting postures on the muscles that attach to the lumbo-pelvic-hip complex with the possible devastating consequence of recurrent lower back pain.

CHAPTER 4
Self-Management of Lower Back Pain

Treatments from qualified professionals, such as doctors, physiotherapists, sports massage therapists, sports therapists, osteopaths or chiropractors, will help to alleviate your acute pain symptoms, although it is likely that you will have to attend more than one session to eradicate your pain completely. However, you should not need treatment for months on end, as it is expensive, time-consuming, and unnecessary. You should therefore be given advice by your chosen professional on a self-management programme. Although you should not rely solely on this book for the management of your lower back problems, it will no doubt assist you in gaining a deeper understanding of the rationale behind these self-help techniques prescribed by your professionals.

4.1.1 General Advice on Self-Management of Lower Back Pain

<u>Stay Active</u>

The traditional management of back pain by resting is now discredited. Your back is designed for movement, and the sooner you get moving and back to ordinary activities, the sooner you will feel better. Simple everyday activities such as walking and gardening can directly ease some of the discomfort by blocking pain signals to the brain. Activity also helps to reduce pain by stretching stiff and tense muscles, ligaments, and joints. However, anything that exacerbates your pain should be avoided, although slight discomfort may have to be accepted when trying to perform normal activities.

When you understand how the body works, it actually makes sense that activity would be better than inactivity to promote healing. From our bones to our soft tissues, our body needs movement and activity to stay in its best condition, because a lack of activity can have several negative effects:

- Muscles can grow stiff and weaken. This explains why muscles tend to feel stiff when you get up in the morning after hours of relative "immobility".
- Soft tissues such as ligaments and tendons can lose their flexibility and become more vulnerable to injury.
- Can be detrimental to the intervertebral discs (please see below).

Without activities, back pain can worsen, which further discourages mobility. In addition, bed rest can be psychologically detrimental to pain sufferers, increasing the likelihood of depression.

Spinal Mobilization Exercises

Our intervertebral discs do not receive a direct blood supply. They derive their oxygen and nutrients from the constant recycling of the disc fluid that occurs with spinal joint movement; i.e., through compression and decompression enabling fluid rich in oxygen and nutrients to be "sucked in" and waste fluid to be "pumped out". The spinal discs are designed for shock absorption and for maintaining spinal flexibility during body movement. A sedentary lifestyle puts constant pressure on the spine and pushes fluid out of the discs which ultimately leads to a reduction in cushioning between the vertebrae, causing decreased mobility and tighter muscles, which can consequently result in back pain. Exercises that increase mobility and relieve tightness and discomfort in your lower back are therefore essential.

Heat Treatment

Heat treatment includes treatments such as using microwavable heat belts or infrared lights (diagram 4.1.1). Many episodes of lower back pain result from strains and overexertions, creating trigger points (section 4.2.4) in the muscles around the lumbo-pelvic-hip complex. This restricts proper circulation and sends pain signals to the brain. Although heat therapy per se will not eradicate trigger points, it can help to provide lower back pain relief through several mechanisms:

- Heat therapy dilates the blood vessels within the muscles surrounding the lumbar spine, enhancing the flow of oxygen and nutrients to the muscles, which helps to heal the damaged tissue.
- Heat stimulates the sensory receptors in the skin, which means that applying heat to the lower back will decrease transmissions of pain signals to the brain and partially relieve the discomfort.
- Heat application makes the soft tissues around the spine more pliable, resulting in a decrease in stiffness, with an increase in flexibility and overall feeling of comfort.

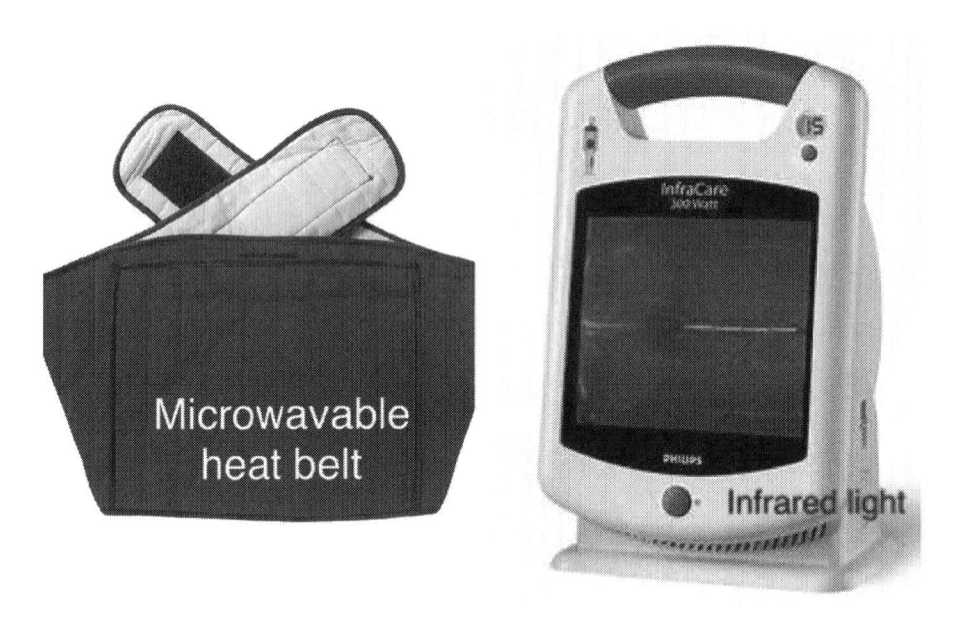

Diagram 4.1.1: Microwavable heat belt and infrared light

Cold Treatment

Cold treatment can be used for short-term pain relief and to relax muscle spasm. As an example of cold treatment, one might apply to the affected area a bag of frozen peas wrapped in a damp towel.

Thermal therapies are appealing because they are simple to apply, inexpensive, non-invasive, and a non-pharmaceutical form of symptomatic relief of lower back pain. From experience, they work best when combined with other treatment modalities, such as physiotherapy, massage and simple exercises (section 4.1.2).

<u>Acupuncture, Painkillers, TENS Machines</u>

From personal experience, the use of these treatments is limited to symptomatic relief, and unless the cause of the problems, such as poor posture or trigger points, are dealt with appropriately, the pain will simply recur.

Acupuncture can help to alleviate back pain by:

- Providing pain relief by stimulating nerves located in muscles and other tissues, as it leads to the release of chemicals such as endorphins and changes the ways pain is processed in the brain and the spinal cord;
- Reducing inflammation;
- Reducing muscle stiffness and improving joint mobility by increasing local microcirculation; and
- Obviating the side effects of using medication.

<u>Trigger-Point Management, Physiotherapy, and Sports Massage</u>

These techniques improve circulation to the tight muscles, get rid of accumulated toxins, and remove and reduce muscle knots and adhesions (section 4.2.3).

4.1.2 Simple Exercises for Alleviation of Acute Lower Back Pain

A natural stimulus for the healing process is active exercise, provided that it is done in a controlled, careful and prescribed manner. While pain often restricts the capability to carry out activities, lack of movement can actually worsen the pain by causing stiffness, weakness and deconditioning. Depending upon your diagnosis and symptoms, your rehabilitation programme may be very different, so it is important to consult appropriate and experienced professionals who can devise a bespoke exercise plan for you and instruct you on the correct forms and techniques.

Generally speaking, the simple activities listed below should help you to quickly decrease your pain. These are important components of your emergency back pain management, as they can alleviate your acute pain, and can be performed many times throughout the day. Please note, however, that these are not corrective exercises (sections 4.2 to 4.5) designed to prevent recurrence in the long term.

Elbow Prop-Up Exercise (Diagram 4.1.2.1)

The prone prop-up exercise should help to alleviate your lower back pain.

Teaching points – lie on your stomach and slowly prop yourself up onto your elbows, causing your lower back to extend back slightly. If your pain worsens in this position, either hold momentarily before progressing or simply return to lying face down and relax for a moment before attempting again. If possible, remain in the propped-up position for a brief moment before slowly returning to your starting position. Perform ten repetitions slowly, and then progress to the following exercise.

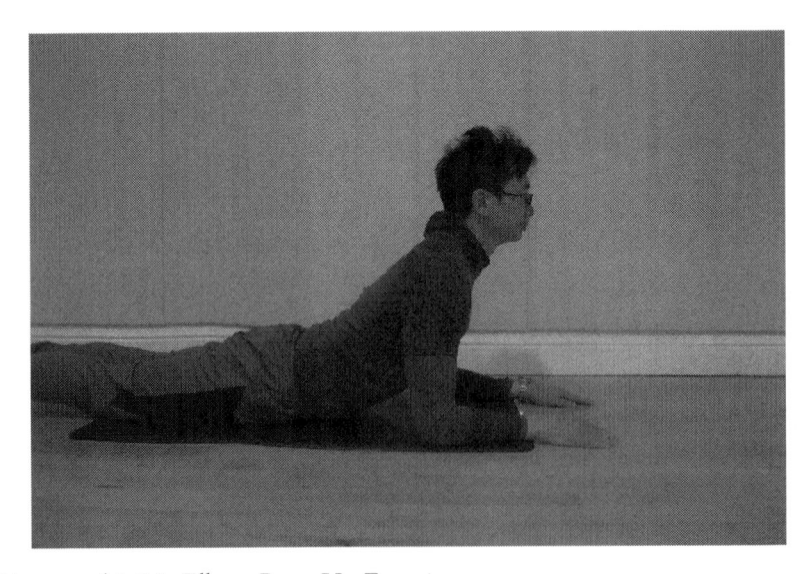

Diagram 4.1.2.1: Elbow Prop-Up Exercise

Press Up with Your Lower Body Remaining on the Floor (Diagram 4.1.2.2)

The objective of this exercise is to restore your normal lumbar lordotic curve.

Teaching points – lie face down with your hands flat on the floor under your shoulders, and then slowly press up so that your upper body extends while your pelvis remains on the floor.

You may not go very far if the pain is too intense. If so, simply slowly lower down and rest for a moment and then press up again. Attempt to go a little further each time. Again, monitor any changes in your symptoms. Perform about ten repetitions, and then relax once again to your starting position.

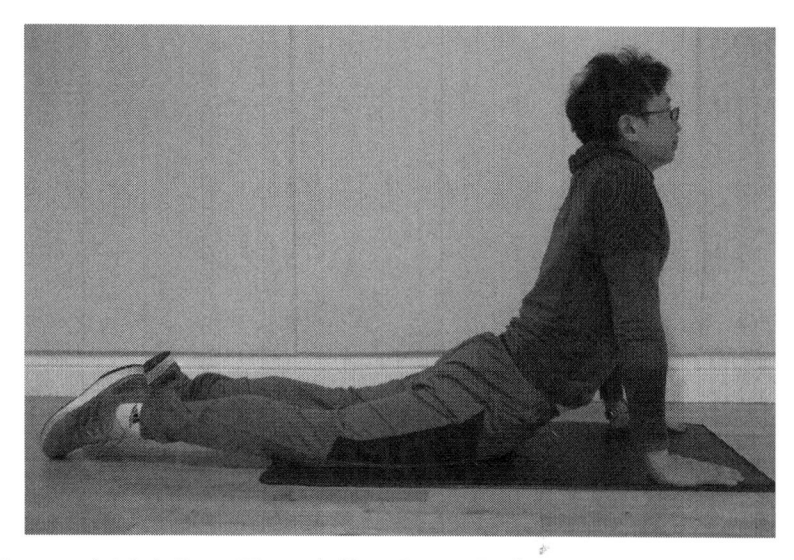

Diagram 4.1.2.2: Press Up with Your Lower Body Remaining on the Floor

Supine spinal twist

This is a spinal rotation exercise while you lie on your back. Although this simple exercise can be very relieving, it can also be associated with the risk of herniated disc, sacroiliac instability, and other injuries because certain conditions might be exacerbated with diagonal mechanical stresses. You are therefore advised to seek professional advice prior to embarking on this exercise.

Teaching points – this simple version involves bending your knees, but with your feet flat on the floor. With your shoulders also flat on the floor, and both arms stretched out to the sides and on the floor for stability, cross your knees over the trunk to one side, then slowly to the other side. You may not be able to take your knees all the way down to the floor at this stage, but going part of the way is acceptable. As you bring your knees over to the side, be aware of your symptoms, and if there is pain, stop immediately.

4.1.3 Identification of the Cause of Your Lower Back Problems

As already mentioned, besides addressing your acute episode of pain, in order to avoid recurrence, it is imperative that you manage your back problem holistically, and the most important first step of this holistic approach is to identify and eradicate the cause of your back problems. Trigger points (section 4.2.4) are implicated in the majority of musculoskeletal pain cases, and if they recur in spite of adequate treatment, you need to identify the contributing factors, such as poor posture, that keep the trigger points active and produce symptoms.

Unlike arthritis, where the pathology can be identified radiographically (using X-rays), musculoskeletal back pain is generally difficult diagnose, as there is no pathology involved and it is often hard to identify the exact cause of the problem.

That said, if you suffer from any form of back pain, you need to seek appropriate professional advice. Please remember that if your back pain lasts for more than six weeks, is constantly intense, or is getting worse, or if you exhibit the symptoms described in section 1.1, you must seek immediate medical attention.

Having established that your lower back pain is of a musculoskeletal nature and is not attributed to serious spinal injury or other illness, before implementing any corrective exercises, an integrated assessment process must be carried out to determine the nature of the dysfunction. This assessment includes (but is not limited to) static and dynamic postural assessments, movement assessments, range-of-motion tests, and muscle strength assessments. These will help to determine which tissues need to be inhibited and lengthened, and which need to be activated and strengthened.

For instance, to check for muscle imbalances, your therapist needs to combine flexibility tests of the global muscles with inner range-holding tests of the postural muscles. An example of a flexibility test is the straight-leg raise test for the hamstrings. You lie on your back with your knees bent. Your therapist takes one leg and straightens it at the knee. If the hamstrings are flexible enough, the leg will raise to about ninety degrees before the hamstrings pull on the lumbar spine. A short hamstring will start to pull on the lumbar spine much earlier.

An example of an inner-range holding test is the prone leg lift for the gluteus maximus. While lying flat on your front, you will be instructed by your therapist to lift one of your thighs a little off the floor. You should be able to feel a strong contraction of the gluteal muscle and be able to hold the static contraction for sixty seconds. If this position places too much strain on the hamstrings or lower back, or if the leg starts shaking, then you are probably unable to recruit the gluteal muscles sufficiently to hold this position. You will feel strain on the hamstrings and lower back (erector spinae), as these are the synergist muscles for hip extension. If your glutes are not firing properly, these synergist muscles for hip extension become overactive.

The above are only examples of what your therapist may use to establish the nature of your muscle imbalances in order that a bespoke corrective exercise programme can be offered. There are other tests for tightness of your hip flexors, piriformis, adductors, and strength of your gluteus medius, and so on. These tests are beyond the scope of this book, as we are only focusing on the self-management protocol of lower back pain.

Lower back pain is complex, and there are often multiple causes for it (section 3.1). The key to managing this pain effectively is accurate assessment. Your therapists should always keep their differential diagnoses in the back of their mind and methodically eliminate each one as they go. The problem is that it is sometimes hard to work out the relationship between cause and effect. It is the proverbial chicken or egg argument: are the muscle imbalances a result of poor posture, or are they the actual cause of the postural dysfunction? For example, your hyperkyphosis may not be a result of poor postural habits, but caused by muscle imbalance of overactive pectorals, possibly due to overtraining your chest muscles in the gym.

If the cause of your lower back pain is your poor posture (chapter 6), it is imperative to get this corrected. This is because your central nervous system gathers and interprets peripheral proprioceptive sensory information in order to execute the appropriate motor response. An individual with poor posture will reinforce these poor habits by delivering improper sensory information to the central nervous system, which can lead to movement compensation. This is because the body will continually adapt in an attempt to produce the functional outcome that is requested by the system. Unfortunately, this adaptability will lead to muscle imbalance, dysfunction and injury, such as musculoskeletal pain. You therefore need to be aware of the "ideal posture" and then consciously train your body so that you can recognize when you are adopting a poor posture. Once you have done this, you should be able to consciously correct it in your everyday routine until the proper posture feels "normal". This can be achieved by learning how to transform your harmful habitual postural patterns into healthy ones; consciously think about your posture, and apply your new knowledge until the new posture and movement patterns become established as the norm. Correcting your posture will feel awkward initially because your body has adapted to sitting and standing in a particular way.

If your back pain is caused by abdominal obesity (chapter 5), you need to get this dealt with so that the associated hyperlordotic posture (section 6.2.1) and anterior pelvic tilt can be reversed.

If your back pain is caused by your flat feet (chapter 7), this needs to be corrected by your podiatrist.

You are reminded that the purpose of this book is not to offer you any diagnosis or medical advice. If you have a recurrent lower back problem, it is imperative that you seek advice from the appropriate professionals. It is impossible to establish a definitive diagnosis without your relevant medical and social histories being noted and thorough assessments being carried out. The advice given in this book is generalized and cannot be substituted for proper professional assistance.

4.1.4 Corrective Exercises for Lower Back Pain

Once you have identified the cause of your musculoskeletal lower back problems, you can start embarking on corrective exercises for the pain. These exercises are advocated by the NASM (National Academy of Sports Medicine). The corrective exercise continuum for the management of lower back pain involves four distinct phases:

- **Inhibitory phase**: This phase involves inhibiting the activity of overactive or tight muscles by using self-myofascial release (section 4.2).
- **Lengthening phase**: Once the overactive muscles have been inhibited, they need to be stretched or lengthened (section 4.3).
- **Activation phase**: This phase involves activation of underactive muscles (section 4.4).
- **Integration phase**—This phase involves the use of dynamic total body exercises to enhance functional capacity. These exercises focus on the synergistic function of the stabilization and mobilization muscles of the body. This involves low load and controlled movement in an ideal posture (section 4.5).

It is important to be aware that tight or overactive muscles not only switch off the antagonist through reciprocal inhibition (section 3.5), but they can also become active in movements that they are not normally associated with. The rationale behind the above continuum is that when you attempt to correct a muscle imbalance, you should always first inhibit the overactive muscles before lengthening them, because trigger points are prone to react to stretching with a defensive tightening. Lengthening tight muscles helps to restore their "normal" length-tension relationship (section 2.6). Furthermore, you cannot effectively strengthen muscles that have trigger points because these fibres are already physiologically contracted. You should therefore activate weakened muscles only after the first two phases of inhibition and lengthening. Please be reminded that if these muscle imbalances are not effectively addressed, the body will be forced into a compensatory position that increases the stress placed on the musculoskeletal system, subsequently leading to lower back pain (section 6.2.8).

4.2 Inhibitory Phase

This phase involves the inhibition of the activity of overactive or tight muscles using self-myofascial release (SMR).

4.2.1 Background

Trigger points are implicated in approximately 75 per cent to 95 per cent of muscular pain cases[6], and inactivity is a major perpetuator. In recent years, technology and automation have reduced the amount of physical activity being undertaken. People are generally more inactive than they used to be, and therefore musculoskeletal conditions—especially neck and back pain—have become more prevalent.

4.2.2 Myofascial Pain Syndrome

This is characterized by chronic pain generated by either fascial constrictions (adhesions) or trigger points ("knots"), which can appear anywhere in the body.

4.2.3 Adhesions of Fascia

Like trigger points, adhesions are a common cause of muscular pain. Adhesions are more about the fascial system than the muscular system.

4.2.3.1 Fascia

Fascia is the connective tissue that wraps and supports our organs, bones and tendons, but it is not just a system of separate coverings; it is actually one continuous structure that exists from head to toe without interruption.

In fact, each part of the entire body is connected to every other part by the fascial system.

4.2.3.2 Myofascia

Where fascia wraps muscles, it is known as myofascia. Myofascia is scaffolding for the muscles, keeping them separate or together when needed for movement. Myofascia surrounds and permeates skeletal muscles. An individual skeletal muscle may be made up of numerous muscle fibres bundled together and wrapped in a connective tissue called the epimysium, which gives the muscle its shape as well as providing a surface against which the surrounding muscles can move. A proportion of this epimysium projects inward to separate the muscle into compartments. Each compartment contains a bundle of muscle fibres known as a fascicle, which is wrapped in connective tissue (perimysium), and each single fibre within the bundle is wrapped in connective tissue called the endomysium.

In a normal healthy state, fascia is viscoelastic and able to stretch and move without restriction. The following factors can cause tightening of this once flexible structure:

- Inflammation
- Traumas and injuries, such as a fall or car accident
- Prolonged poor postural habits
- Lack of flexibility due to prolonged sitting or standing
- Long-term psychological stresses
- Repetitive muscle strain injuries.

Microscopically, myofascia resembles a fishnet and is well organized and very flexible in a healthy state. However, during repair processes, it forms scar tissues, and when it gets stuck to other tissues, your muscles may feel as if they have been tied in knots, which can restrict their normal range of movements. Myofascia is like a complete bodysuit; it is continuous, and therefore damage to an area of fascia can affect other distant areas of your body, creating problems far away from the adhesion through compensation patterns, which can potentially affect your posture and movements. These changes to the fascial system adversely affect the comfort and function of the body by exerting excessive pressure, affecting your flexibility and stability, and causing all kinds of pain symptoms.

Physiology of Fascial Repair

There is an important substance in fascia called ground substance. When you are young and healthy, this substance is gelatinous, but as you get older, biochemical and mechanical traumas transform the texture of this ground substance, from soft and flexible to thick and gluey, causing tightening of myofascia, making it more difficult for nutrients to move through the myofascial network and harder for waste to be removed. The good news is that this tightening of ground substance is reversible.

4.2.3.3 Treatment of Adhesion Using Self Myofascial Release (SMR)

SMR can directly change and improve the health of fascia. The objective of SMR is to break up scar tissue, increase circulation, and help to remove toxic metabolic waste that has been restricted by the contracted tissue. Deep tissue massage carried out by your therapist can be performed at home by yourself, using devices such as foam rollers.

4.2.4 Trigger Points

Besides the aforementioned muscle tightness being caused by the formation of scar tissue during the repair processes of myofascia, trigger points that are formed within muscles can also make muscles tight and restrict their movements. Trigger points typically develop in the centre of the muscle belly where the motor endplate (section 2.5) is located. In fact, trigger points can occur anywhere in any muscle and in any layer of any muscle, and each muscle layer can have multiple trigger points (section 4.2.4.5 below).

The term trigger point was developed in 1942 by Dr Janet Travell. Some authors consider a trigger point to be just another name for fascial adhesion, but according to Travell and Simons[7] it is defined as "a highly irritable localized spot of exquisite tenderness in a nodule in a palpable taut band of muscle tissue". Trigger points are in fact, a small patch of tightly contracted muscle, an isolated "spasm" affecting just an individual myofibril.

A Practical Guide to the Self-Management of Lower Back Pain

The body's neuromuscular system can easily be adversely affected by poor posture, repetitive muscle strain or dysfunctional movements. These mechanically stressful actions are recognized as an injury by the body, initiating a repair process called the **cumulative injury cycle** (section 6.2.8), which follows a pathway of inflammation and the development of fascial adhesions and trigger points that can lead to altered neuromuscular control and muscle imbalance caused by reduction in muscular elasticity. SMR focuses on alleviating these adhesions and trigger points to restore optimal muscle function.

Trigger points can also be considered to be part of our protective mechanism. Any change in spinal biomechanics over time can manifest as areas of tight muscles; because trigger points make the host muscles weak (weak because these fibres are already contracted and cannot contribute to further contraction), they are a useful mechanism for rapidly switching off muscle power around an injury. This is essential if, say, there is a fracture. They are an important part of our defend, protect, and repair mechanism, and the nervous system uses trigger points to accomplish this objective.

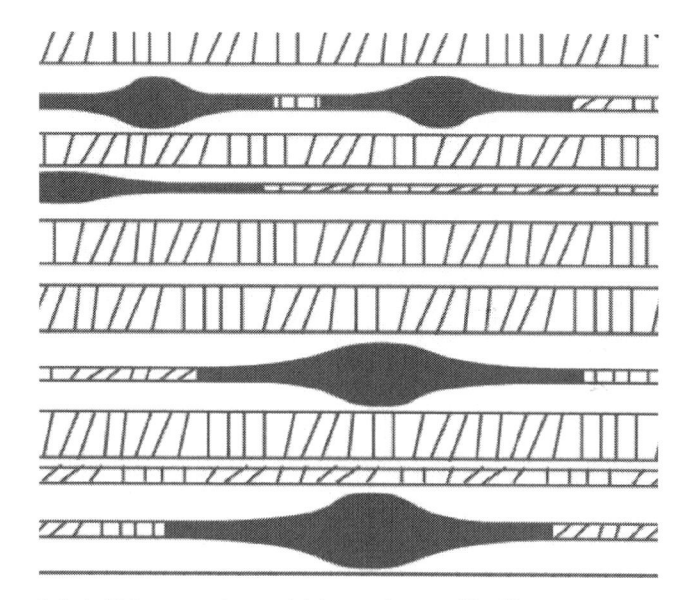

Diagram 4.2.4: Trigger points within each myofibril[8]

Unlike acupuncture points or meridians, trigger points can be felt with your fingers. Give it a try by running your finger along your calf muscles; you should be able to locate numerous tender trigger points there. They are actually small contraction knots within muscle fibres that "refuse" to release. Apart from keeping the muscle fibre involved tight and weak, these tight areas restrict blood and lymphatic circulation in the immediate vicinity, resulting in accumulation of metabolic by-products and deprivation of oxygen and nutrients. This crisis of energy produces sensitizing substances that can cause pain. For example, **bradykinin** is known to activate and sensitize muscle pain receptors (nociceptors).

Physiology of Trigger Points

Muscles with trigger points manifest in the region where sarcomeres and motor endplates become overactive. Essentially, the actin and myosin myofilaments sitting within a taught band stop sliding over one another.

When the nerve impulse arrives at the motor endplate, neurotransmitter acetylcholine is released causing calcium to be released from the sarcoplasmic reticulum (SR) and the muscle fibre involved to contract (section 2.5). Normally, when contraction of the muscle fibre ceases, the motor endplate stops releasing acetylcholine and the "calcium pump" in the SR recycles calcium back into the SR.

When there is an excessive motor endplate release of acetylcholine, surplus calcium can be released by the SR, causing a maximal contracture of a segment of muscle, leading to maximal energy demand and impairment of local circulation. As a result of this deprivation of fuel and oxygen, the calcium pump is unable to return calcium back into the SR and the muscle fibre maintains its contraction (trigger point). This vicious circle is self-perpetuating unless there is some form of intervention, such as SMR. Furthermore, the attachment sites of these tight muscle fibres can also become tender as they are stressed by the contraction in the centre of the fibre, causing formation of attachment trigger points (section 4.2.4.5).

Problems with Chronic Back Pain

Although the acute phase of musculoskeletal back pain typically subsides within one week or so even without intervention, many suffer from recurrent symptoms. This is because without treatment, trigger points simply turn latent and can be reactivated with the slightest overload, for example by twisting or bending awkwardly. It is therefore important to not simply address the acute episode of back pain, but to manage it by identifying the causes of functional deficiencies, and then to deal with the problems holistically using the corrective exercise continuum (section 4.1.4).

4.2.4.1 Symptoms of Trigger Points

Trigger points often cause symptoms that mimic common medical conditions. This is because muscles that have been shortened and enlarged by trigger points frequently compress nearby nerves, and those that pass through a muscle are particularly vulnerable. This can cause distortion of the electrical signals that travel along these nerves, resulting in altered sensations, including numbness, dizziness, itchiness, burning, prickling, heat, or hypersensitivity in the areas supplied by the nerve. Trigger points can also cause a muscle to restrict blood flow in an artery, making a distant body part feel cold.

Trigger points are known to cause headaches, neck pain, and lower back pain, and many types of joint pain are often mistakenly ascribed to arthritis, tendonitis, bursitis, or ligament injury. They can cause problems as diverse as earache, vertigo, dizziness, nausea, heartburn, false anginal pain, tennis/golfer's elbow, tension headache, temporomandibular joint symptoms, facial pain, sinus pain, and toothache. They can be responsible for chronic pain and disability that seem to have no means of relief, which can ultimately result in depression. They are also treatable causes of range of motion loss (trigger points affect movement by keeping muscles short and stiff), muscle weakness, pain, and other symptoms often blamed on old age.

Osteoarthritis may be minimized if related trigger points are promptly treated. Therefore, any arthritis treatment and prevention programme should include treatment of the related trigger points, as this will improve neuromuscular function and coordination and thus prevent or hinder the progression of osteoarthritis.

4.2.4.2 Prevalence of Trigger Points

We all have trigger points; the question is the degree to which they affect us. There are over seven hundred muscles in our bodies, and any one of these muscle can develop trigger points which can refer pain elsewhere. Therefore, working on the area where you feel symptoms may not give you relief. More often than not, doctors tend to look at the place that hurts rather than find the source of the pain. This is because although a muscle is an important tissue, no medical speciality claims it. Muscle tissue is complex and vulnerable to dysfunction, and it is the primary target of wear and tear through daily activities. Nevertheless, it is the bones, joints, and nerves on which doctors usually concentrate their attention.

Trigger points are so common that even children and babies have them. They can exist indefinitely in a latent state until intervention occurs. These trigger points accumulate over a lifetime and appear to be the main cause of stiff joints and the restriction of a range of movements. They can also keep muscles out of balance, causing joints to click during function. A typical example of this would be trigger points in the vastus lateralis and the vastus medialis of the quadriceps group of muscles. These muscles attach to the anterior upper tibia via the patella tendon. Trigger points in these muscles cause muscular imbalance, leading to abnormal tracking of the patella within the femoral trochlea. When the patella is not properly aligned within the femoral trochlea, the stress per unit area on the patella cartilage increases as a result of a smaller contact area between the patella and the trochlea; this ultimately leads to the knee joint clicking during function and, eventually, osteoarthritis.

4.2.4.3 Characteristics of Trigger Points

Trigger points, either active or latent, are easy to locate because they are always very painful when pressed on. Please note that trigger points are not the same as muscle spasms; a spasm involves a violent contraction of the entire muscle, which can be relaxed in a matter of minutes. Trigger points are contractions within a muscle fibre (myofibril) that cannot be released without treatment.

It is important to realize that the level of pain depends more on the degree of trigger point irritability than the size of the muscle. Trigger points in the tiniest muscle, such as the piriformis (section 4.3.2.5) of the glutes, can cause crippling lower back pain.

The problem is that trigger points can refer pain to another site. Once you know where to look, however, they are easily located by touch and deactivated through SMR. The predictable referral patterns of various trigger points within various muscles are well documented, and the referral maps for these are widely available. When you press on a trigger point, you should often be able to feel the pain spreading to the predictable referral site. For instance, when you press on a trigger point in the upper trapezius, you should be able to feel the referral pain travelling up your neck. This is not a textbook on trigger points, and it is beyond the scope of this book to elaborate on the referral patterns of all the common trigger points in the body.

Pain from the lower back can originate from trigger points in your gluteal muscles—especially the piriformis (section 4.3.2.5) and the glute medius (section 4.2.6.6). The reverse is also true; trigger points in the lower back often refer pain down to the buttocks and hips. Trigger points in the superficial spinal muscles (e.g. erector spinae, section 4.2.6.4) cause a more diffuse type of pain than the trigger points in the deep spinal muscles (e.g. multifidus). The superficial spinal muscles are particularly vulnerable when you do anything strenuous while bending to one side; lifting something this way puts the full load on just one half of the back, effectively doubling the strain.

Trigger points typically cause pain on the same side of the body. Rarely do they send pain to the opposite side. The most reliable criterion for detecting a trigger point is its extreme tenderness. Simply seek the spot along the muscle that hurts the most when you press on it.

When investigating back pain, trigger points should be at the top of the list, because it has been estimated that in 75 to 95 per cent of muscular pain cases, myofascial trigger points are a primary cause. Unfortunately, doctors may not be fully aware of trigger points. Misdiagnosis of such a "simple" source of musculoskeletal problems can lead to unnecessary invasive treatment when such problems are wrongly ascribed as osteoarthritis. That said, although trigger points are frequently implicated in musculoskeletal pain, there could be underlying pathology, and you should seek medical advice if you suffer from back pain.

Even when back pain is due to genuine problems in your spine, trigger points may still be causing a major part of your pain. Doctors Janet Travell and David Simons, the foremost authorities on myofascial pain, believe that trigger points may actually be the root cause of many genuine spinal problems, such as a prolapsed or herniated disc, because trigger points keep the host muscles short and tight. This can be the ultimate source of disc compression and spinal nerve impingement.

4.2.4.4 Causes of Trigger Points

There are numerous causes of trigger points. Listed below are just some more common examples.

- **Mechanical stressors:** These stressors include muscle trauma from car accidents, falls, and sports- and work-related injuries. Other causes include paradoxical breathing, repetitive movement, body disproportion, muscle abuse, postural dysfunction, and muscle strain or sitting improperly for long periods. For example, prolonged sitting and a sedentary lifestyle are strong perpetuators of trigger points, because muscles need to work in order to stay healthy. Keeping muscles inactive for a prolonged period of time encourages them to stiffen and grow weak, and weakness is often a contributory factor in the pathogenesis of myofascial trigger points, because your body overcompensates for the weakness in the muscle by overstimulating the motor endplate.
- **Metabolic factors:** These include impairment to the energy metabolism, certain vitamin and mineral deficiencies, and metabolic disorders.

- **Environmental factors:** These include allergies, pollution, medications, trauma, and infections.
- **Psychological factors:** These include chronic stress and anxiety.

4.2.4.5 Types of Trigger Points

- Primary or central trigger points always exist in the centre of the muscle belly, where the motor endplate (section 2.5) enters the muscle. The problem is that the fibres do not always run from end to end in a muscle, because the orientation of the fibres in muscles varies, depending on their role. In muscles that are designed for speed, the fibres are parallel, running straight from end to end, and their trigger points are easily found in the middle of the muscle belly. However, muscles made for power will have fibres running diagonally (such as in multipennate muscles, e.g., the deltoid) at some angles to its length. Since trigger points may be found in the centre of each individual fibre, they may be situated anywhere along the muscle.

- Satellite or secondary trigger points are created in response to the primary ones in neighbouring muscles that lie within the referral pain zone. Muscles do not operate in isolation (section 3.3.2.3), and this is why the development of primary trigger points in one area of the body can lead to satellite points distally. They often resolve once the primary point has been deactivated.

- Attachment trigger points are found where the tendon of the muscle inserts into the bone. For instance, you can typically find attachment trigger points of the gluteus medius where it attaches to the greater trochanter of the femur.

- Diffuse trigger points can be found where multiple satellite points exist secondary to multiple primary trigger points. These are often found where there is a severe postural deformity, such as in scoliosis (section 6.2.3).

- Inactive or latent trigger points are symptomless and do not elicit a referred pain pathway. They do, however, increase muscle stiffness, and these points are prevalent in those with a sedentary lifestyle. They can be reactivated with the slightest overload, such as twisting and bending. Latent trigger points are the main cause of stiff joints and the restriction of a range of movements due to muscle tightness and weakness of the host muscle. They can also keep muscles out of balance, causing joints to click during function, and can potentially lead to osteoarthritis.

- Active trigger points can be either primary or satellite. They are tender to palpation and elicit a referred pain pattern. Active trigger points usually refer pain locally and/or to distant areas of the body. Common patterns have been identified, but these referral patterns do not necessarily conform to the nerve pathways. As the majority of trigger points are not located where you feel symptoms, treating the painful area will not provide relief. To complicate the situation further, they can also manifest in secondary muscles or as satellite trigger points in and around the vicinity of the primary site.

4.2.4.6 Treatment of Trigger Points Using Self Myofascial Release (SMR)

Simply rubbing the surface of the skin, using a vibrating massager or applying heat will not release a trigger point. Sufficiently deep sustained pressure to the "knotted-up area" is required.

SMR will not only improve the health of myofascia by breaking up the scar tissues, it can also break into the chemical and neurological feedback loop that maintains the trigger points. Furthermore, it increases circulation, helps to remove toxic metabolic waste that has been restricted by the contracted tissue, and directly stretches the trigger point's knotted muscle fibres. Massage should be deep and in one direction only (it is not advisable to rub the trigger points to and fro, table 4.2.6.2), and the pace should be slow because the aim is to deactivate overactive tissue, and nothing should be done to make the tissue more excited.

4.2.4.7 Physiology of SMR

The science behind SMR is autogenic inhibition, and this involves the interplay between the two neural receptors, muscle spindles, and the Golgi tendon organs (GTO) that are found in skeletal muscles.

Muscle spindles respond to a change and rate of muscle lengthening/stretching by causing the muscle involved to contract. This is a protective mechanism (stretch reflex) in order to prevent a muscle tear when you stretch it too far.

The GTOs are located in the tendons connecting the muscle to bone, and when the rate of increase of muscle tension is increased (caused by excessive muscle contraction), they respond by causing the muscle to relax. When a change in tension is maintained at an adequate intensity and duration, the GTO will inhibit the activity of the muscle spindle, which will in turn reduce trigger point activity. In simpler terms, when the pressure of the body against a trigger point tool, such as a foam roller or a trigger point ball, is sustained on the trigger point, the GTO will "turn off" the muscle spindle activity, allowing the muscle fibres to stretch, unknot, and realign.

4.2.4.8 How Long Does It Take to Get Relief from Trigger Points?

The length of time it takes to release a trigger point depends on several factors. Type 1 postural fibres (section 2.3) tend to respond to stress or overuse by shortening. A trigger point in a muscle with a high percentage of type 1 fibres may take a few weeks or even months to respond to treatment. A trigger point in a muscle with a high percentage of type 2 fibres may respond more rapidly, usually within a week or two.

You may ask, why you would bother if it takes over a week to release trigger points, when your acute back pain may subside after a week or so anyway. Remember that the pain subsides without treatment only because the trigger points implicated in the back pain have turned latent, and they can be reactivated very easily with the slightest overload such as awkwardly twisting or bending your torso. The purpose of working on these trigger points is not just to relieve the acute pain, but to prevent recurrence.

Other factors include the number of trigger points you have, how regularly you can administer or receive treatment, and how long you have had the trigger points. Chronic trigger points have made pathways in the nervous system that tend to reinforce and perpetuate them[9]. Acute lower back pain responds very well to SMR. However, long-term or recurrent lower back disorders can become more complicated, because they often involve many more muscle groups and multiple trigger point interactions.

Furthermore, are you dealing only with a satellite trigger points (section 4.2.4.5) rather than identifying and treating the primary ones? How effective are you in eradicating the perpetuating factors of the trigger points in the first place, such as postural dysfunction (chapter 6), flat feet (chapter 7) or repetitive movement patterns? It must be emphasized that poor posture is a powerful perpetuator of myofascial trigger points. This is because postural muscles tend to have a greater percentage of type 1 fibres and are more resistant to treatment.

Another preventable perpetuating factor is inappropriate exercises. You cannot effectively strengthen muscles that have trigger points, because individual muscle fibres affected by trigger points are already contracted and cannot contribute to the contraction of the whole muscle. The muscle must therefore first be brought to a healthy state prior to strengthening. Overdoing a good exercise can be detrimental, and overstretching a muscle can cause reactive shortening.

If the primary trigger points are not properly treated and perpetuating factors are not brought under control, trigger points can spread. If the trigger point still does not deactivate after the third application, it may be a satellite point, and in that case you need to identify the location of the primary point and deactivate it first.

You may be tempted to discontinue working on the trigger point the moment it stops actively referring pain. However, please remember that if the trigger point still hurts when you press on it, you have only soothed it into a latent state which can be easily reactivated with the slightest overload or awkward bending.

From a practical point of view, even if you are able to have your trigger point or the source of pain identified by your therapist, it is both costly and time-consuming to pay someone to completely release all the primary, latent, and satellite myofascial trigger points you may have in your body. Trigger points need to be worked on daily using a technique that will apply the pinpoint pressure that is required. SMR is beneficial because you can perform this at home, at work, or in the gym as often as you like.

If you use a foam roller regularly, you should do so after a warm-up but before dynamic stretching (section 5.6.1), thus improving the tissue's ability to lengthen during stretching activities. You should also do SMR at the end of your exercise session, prior to static stretching.

4.2.5 The Relationship between Fibromyalgia (FM) and Trigger Points

This is not a medical textbook but FM is worth mentioning briefly. FM is the term given to a family of illnesses that have in common central nervous system sensitisation and chronic diffuse systemic pain. It is systemic and not local. Although unexplained, FM might be a clearer neurological disease.

Myofascial pain syndrome and FM are both characterized by hypersensitive spots in various parts of the body. With FM, these spots are called tender points, which differ from trigger points. A trigger point needs firm pressure to elicit pain while a tender point is so painful that it can hardly be touched. In addition, unlike trigger points that refer pain elsewhere, tender points cause only local pain. That said, genuine FM sufferers often have both types of points, and trigger points are one of the main factors generating and perpetuating FM pain and other symptoms, irrespective of what initiated the FM in the first place. The FM amplifies the pain and other symptoms.

Trigger points have extreme tenderness which always reveals their location. They can always be felt with the fingers. People with FM ordinarily hurt all over and often can hardly bear to be touched. Tender points are typically present almost everywhere, and are not limited to muscle tissues. Furthermore, muscles with trigger points feel firm while the muscles of FM sufferers are soft and doughy.

Muscles with trigger points stiffen the joints and inhibit your range of movement. In FM, the joints are loose, or even hypermobile. Depression can come with both conditions but people with myofascial pain can generally get on with life. People with FM are frequently overwhelmed by extreme fatigue and are unable to move without experiencing agonizing pain. SMR will have no effect on FM.

4.2.6 Practical Advice on Self Myofascial Release (Table 4.2.6.2)

SMR not only will improve the health of the myofascia by breaking up the scar tissues, but also can break into the chemical and neurological feedback loop that maintains the trigger points. You will be introduced next to the safe and effective ways to perform these procedures.

4.2.6.1 The Ten-Second Press Test[10]

When you feel a lump or tightness in a muscle tissue and it is painful, how can you be sure that this is a trigger point and it is safe to perform SMR on it?

You may perform the ten-second press test by applying progressive downward pressure on the area of discomfort, using either your finger or a small trigger point ball (see later). Continue applying the pressure until the pain has reached seven out of ten (ten being the most unbearable level of pain), and maintain this constant pressure for ten seconds.

- If the pain increases, this signifies inflammation, and the pressure must be removed immediately because SMR is inappropriate in this situation.
- If the pain remains constant, this indicates that there is neither inflammation nor a trigger point, and the pain may be due to fascial adhesion (section 4.2.3).
- If the pain decreases, this signifies the presence of a trigger point that is beginning to release in response to the localized deep pressure (section 4.2.4.7).

Deep Stroking Massage	Ischemic Compression Using Static Pressure
Rather than sliding your fingers across the skin, move the skin with your fingers. This enhances blood and lymphatic circulation more effectively. Furthermore, intermittent discomfort (aim for 7/10) is easier to tolerate than continuous pain.	As long as you can tolerate the continuous pain, slowly roll to the targeted area until you find the most tender spot. Hold on to that spot while relaxing the targeted area until the discomfort subsides (between thirty and ninety seconds). Relax and keep on breathing normally.
Massage of a given trigger point should be relatively brief, preferably no more than thirty seconds. Trigger points often release on their own when they receive frequent daily treatment. Treatment failures are usually the result of being too aggressive, treating the wrong spot, or not addressing the perpetuating factors.	A word of warning: please be careful, as overenthusiastic use of hard tools can result in bruising of the skin and deeper tissues, including muscles and nerves, and this is obviously counterproductive.
Perform foam rolling in one direction only, towards your heart, to facilitate lymphatic drainage and avoid damaging the one-way valves of the veins.	This should be repeated a few times a day.
Perform the massage slowly as you do not want to "activate" the muscle, you want to "inhibit" it.	For chronic and stubborn trigger points that refuse to release, typically those on postural muscles with type 1 fibres, an alternative method may be preferred: Apply constant and direct pressure (pain 7/10) for five seconds, and then release the pressure whilst maintaining skin contact for two seconds. Reapply progressive pressure until the pain reaches a level of 7/10, hold for five seconds, and then release for two seconds again. Repeat the process several times until there is a reduction of pain or until two minutes have passed with no change in pain levels.
Limit yourself to eight to ten strokes per trigger point at least five times daily.	It is advisable to listen to music whilst you perform SMR, as this relaxes you and takes your mind off the pain that you may experience.

Table 4.2.6.2: General Treatment Guidelines for Trigger Points

Tools That Can Be Used

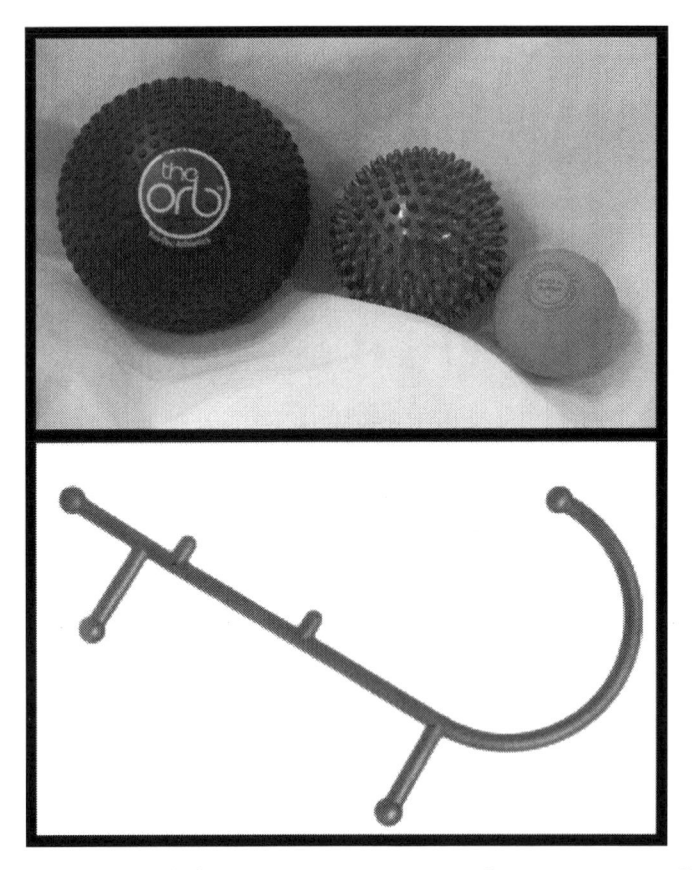

Diagram 4.2.6.2: Tools for SMR; Various Types of Trigger Point Balls on the Top and Theracane on the Bottom

Remember: trigger points often refer pain elsewhere and you may not find the real cause of your lower back pain if you concentrate only on your lower back. It is worth noting that trigger points in the buttocks muscles are a frequent cause of lower back pain (section 4.2.6.6). The reverse is also true; trigger points in the lower back often refer pain down to the buttocks and hips.

4.2.6.3 SMR of Deep Spinal Muscles

Examples of deep spinal muscles are the rotators and multifidus (section 3.3.2).

Common Symptoms

Trigger points in the multifidus often cause sharp pain in the lower back and restrict your movement in all directions. Your back will feel stiff and it will be difficult for you to turn your torso.

Functional Anatomy of the Multifidus

The multifidus is a series of small muscles that travel up the length of the spine. They lie on each side of the spinous processes of the lumbar vertebrae. While the erector spinae move the spine as a whole, the multifidi provide segmental stability by orienting adjacent vertebrae to each other.

> *Origin* - posterior sacrum
>
> *Insertion* - spinous process of vertebrae (except C1), two to four bones above origin

A common cause for formation of trigger points in these deep spinal muscles is poor work ergonomics, such as sitting sideways at the computer or sitting with a twisted posture for a prolonged period of time. These deep spinal muscles, being individually quite small, are particularly vulnerable to sudden overload and repetitive movements. This is particularly relevant when the abdominal core is weak and these small muscles have to work beyond their endurance to compensate.

Teaching points - deep massage right beside the spine with a trigger point ball, using short, slow strokes is beneficial but make sure that you are not pressing directly on the vertebrae.

Simply place the ball on your back in the desired area and slowly roll along the length of the muscle (either against the floor or a wall) until you find the painful spot. Then hold on to it for thirty to forty-five seconds until the pain diminishes. If you are lying on the floor, it is beneficial to place a foam roller below your upper back so that you can use it as a "wheel" to glide along the floor whilst the trigger point ball is actually working on the trigger points on your lower back (Diagram 4.2.6.4). You will have to reposition yourself and the ball a couple of times to work on multiple trigger points.

To prevent back problems from the deep spinal muscles, besides strengthening your abdominal core (section 4.4.3), you need to improve your work ergonomics and avoid twisting.

4.2.6.4 SMR of Erector Spinae

Common Symptoms

Trigger points in the superficial spinal muscles cause a more diffuse type of pain than those in the deep spinal counterparts.

Functional Anatomy

The erector spinae actually consists of three muscle groups running vertically up both sides of the vertebral column—the iliocostalis, longissimus, and spinalis—The iliocostalis is the most lateral muscle group, the longissimus is the intermediate muscle group, and the spinalis is the medial muscle group, adjacent to the spinal column. These muscles function to maintain your spine in an upright position, extend your spine, and provide lateral flexion.

Origin

- Posterior crest of the ilium
- Lower posterior surface of the sacrum
- Lower seven ribs
- Spinous processes of T9-L5
- Transverse processes of T1-12.

Insertion

- Angles of the ribs
- Transverse processes of all vertebrae
- Base of the skull.

Causes of Erector Spinae Trigger Points

The lumbar erector spinae are typically tight in individuals with hyperlordosis as a result of the anterior tilting of the pelvis (section 6.2.1).

Interestingly, pain from the iliocostalis can cause referred pain that can mimic angina, appendicitis, and other visceral conditions. Persistent stiffness in the back can be a sign of latent trigger points in the absence of any pain. These latent trigger points can be reactivated with the slightest stress or strain, such as awkward twisting and turning. These superficial spinal muscles are vulnerable to the formation of trigger points due to prolonged immobility, a sedentary lifestyle, or inappropriate lifting movements. This is particularly true when you lift heavy items from the floor while bending to one side because you put the full load on just one half of your back, effectively doubling the strain on the muscle.

Teaching points - owing to the anatomy of this muscle, it is easy to carry out self-myofascial release with a trigger point ball (a tennis ball is too soft to produce deep, sustained pressure on the trigger points in these muscles).

You can either stand or lie on the floor, similar to the massage of the multifidus. Place the ball on your back in the desired area, and then slowly roll up and down along the length of the muscle until you find the painful spot. Again, place a foam roller below your upper back to assist you in gliding up and down along the floor whilst the lacrosse ball is actually doing the work on the muscle itself (diagram 4.2.6.4). As soon as you find a tender area along the muscle, hold on to it for thirty seconds until the pain diminishes. While you are massaging along the muscle, you will have to reposition yourself and the ball a couple of times or you will not be able to cover your entire lower back.

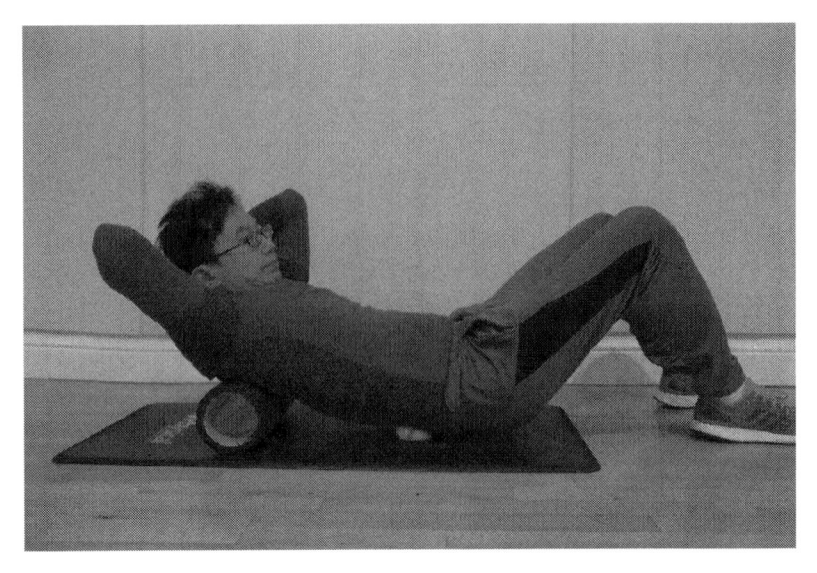

Diagram 4.2.6.4: SMR of the Erector Spinae with a Trigger Point Ball

4.2.6.5 SMR of the Quadratus Lumborum (QL)

Functional Anatomy

The quadratus lumborum (QL) is a small and hidden muscle group of the posterior abdominal wall, but it plays a prominent role in our normal body mechanics by contributing to pelvic stabilization, movement of the spine, and maintenance of an upright posture; thus, it is considered to be one of the core muscles.

It is a muscle of the posterior abdominal wall originating from the posterior third of the iliac crest, and it is attached to the transverse processes of the upper four lumbar vertebrae to the 12th rib. All the fibres together give the muscle a rectangular appearance.

- **Concentric Functions** (section 5.6.7): Unilateral (single-side) contraction causes lateral flexion (sideways bending) of the spine and bilateral (double-sided) contraction causes extension (backward bending) of the lumbar spine.
- **Eccentric and Isometric Functions:** Dynamically stabilizes the lumbo-pelvic-hip complex.

Pathology

Overuse and strain of the QL are major causes of musculoskeletal lower back pain. Furthermore, they can contribute to stress in the sacroiliac joint by pulling it out of alignment (chapter 8).

Characteristics and Symptoms of Lower Back Pain Caused by the QL

Since there can be many reasons for lower back pain (chapter 1), it is essential to distinguish one symptom from another in order to obtain the appropriate treatment.

- Back pain that worsens with prolonged sitting, and when transitioning from sitting to standing.
- The pain can radiate towards the pelvic, gluteal, and groin regions.
- If you have a sudden attack of unilateral lower back pain, perhaps a short while after lifting something heavy, then you may have strained your QL, which is particularly vulnerable if you have bent over while letting your lower back arch forward. There may be excruciating lower back pain in an unsupported, upright position, and movement of the spine is usually restricted. Often, it is difficult to roll from side to side in bed, and sufferers can experience great difficulties in getting out of bed in the morning.
- Since the QL is an auxiliary respiratory muscle through its attachment to the 12th rib, coughing and sneezing can cause pain as it contracts to stabilize the ribcage.

QL trigger points are considered to be the "masters of lower back pain", especially in those cases where the pain is so severe that you cannot stand up.

Causes of QL Trigger Points

- Overuse and strain: Any activity, such as lifting, that involves bending and twisting at the waist. This is because when you twist your torso, the QL on the side you are twisting towards contracts, along with the erector spinae and internal obliques on the same side, and the external obliques on the opposite side. If you lean over and twist at the same time, this puts your QL on the side you are twisting towards on "double duty". You request your QL to both rotate your torso and extend your back while in a mechanically disadvantageous position (assuming you have allowed your lower back to flex forward, as the majority do when bending over).

- A sedentary lifestyle: The QL is one of the few muscles that gets overused even when you are sitting. This is because prolonged sitting causes tightness and weakening of the hip flexor (iliopsoas) muscles, which in turn inhibits the antagonists, the glutes, through reciprocal inhibition (section 3.5). The glutes are responsible for hip extension and pelvic stabilization, and their weaknesses lead to their action being compensated for by the QL (see synergistic dominance in section 3.6), causing the QL to overwork and prompting the formation of trigger points. The gluteal (especially the gluteus medius) and quadratus muscles work together, and they are usually afflicted by trigger points at the same time.
- Trauma: This includes car accidents and any other incidents that cause direct damage to the QL.
- Bending over: This includes bending over whilst standing to put on your pants or socks. You are especially prone to injury if your foot gets entangled and you lose your balance.
- A genetically short leg: This can cause a lateral tilt in the pelvis, forcing the QL to overwork to stabilize the pelvis.
- Core dysfunction (section 3.3)
- Sleeping on a soft mattress that sags (section 9.3): This may activate or reactivate QL trigger points by placing the muscle in a shortened or stretched position for an extended period.

The primary antagonist to each QL muscle is the contralateral QL muscle. Thus, if one muscle develops trigger point activity, the muscle on the other side will become overloaded and also develop trigger points. Treatment should always address the trigger points in both QLs even if the pain is limited to one side only.

Associated Trigger Points

Effective treatment of the QL trigger points will also need to address the associated trigger points in other muscle groups. Pain from the QL trigger point can be referred to all the gluteal muscles and activate the satellite trigger points there. Furthermore, as both the QL and hip flexors share the function of stabilizing the lumbar spine, trigger point-induced weakness in one of the muscle groups tends to overload the other muscle group and cause secondary trigger points to develop within it.

How Can You Release QL Trigger Points?

If the QL is causing pain, there are likely to be trigger points in several places, especially near the attachments at the pelvis and bottom ribs.

From personal experience, the best tools to use are a trigger point ball or a Thera Cane (section 4.2.4.6). You can either stand against a wall or lie on your back and roll the ball against the trigger points where you can feel the pain. Hold on to the painful area until the pain dissipates.

Prevention: Posture, Lifting Technique, and Strength

QL pain will recur unless you stop sitting all day and vary your posture as you sit. Strengthen your QL so that it can handle the demands you place upon it, and stop misusing your back when you lift objects. It is also important not to sit with your legs crossed, as this places too much strain on the QL on one side.

As for misusing your QL, you also need to learn to lift objects properly by not relying solely on your lower back. Lift heavy objects by squatting down low and using your quadriceps and glutes to return to the standing position. Engage your core (section 4.4.2.3) and maintain a neutral spine the whole time. Lift lighter objects the same way, or by using the golfer's pick-up, planting one leg and allowing the other to lift off the ground behind you as you lean over.

4.2.6.6 SMR of Gluteal Muscles

<u>Gluteus Maximus</u>

Functional Anatomy

The gluteus maximus is the most superficial of the gluteal musculature, and it forms the surface anatomy of the gluteal region. It is the most powerful hip extensor and abductor, and it also supports and stabilizes the pelvis.

It originates from the sacrum, coccyx, and the iliac crest and inserts at the gluteal tuberosity of the femur and the iliotibial band (ITB), a strong fibrous band at the outside of the thigh inserting at the lateral condyle at the tibia.

Sitting for too long activates trigger points in the gluteus maximus, which can refer pain to your lower back. With your glute being tight (often with your hamstrings being tight due to prolonged sitting), you may no longer be able to bend over and touch your toes.

Prevention

Avoid prolonged sitting as this can encourage latent trigger points to develop, which makes the muscle stiff. The pressure from sitting also restricts normal circulation to the gluteal muscles.

Treatment

Sitting on a trigger point ball or foam roller, roll slowly with a deep stroke across the trigger point. This is preferable to static pressure.

Gluteus Medius

Although trigger points in the gluteus medius are commonly implicated in lower back pain, its involvement is often overlooked. Pain from trigger points in the gluteus medius is felt in the lower back, just above and below the beltline, occasionally extending into the buttocks and hip areas. You may also feel pain when walking or sleeping on your side.

Functional Anatomy

The gluteus medius runs from your iliac crest to the greater trochanter of the femur, deep to (covered by) the gluteus maximus. Anterior fibres are responsible for abduction (moving the leg away from the midline) and internal hip rotation, and posterior fibres are responsible for extension and external hip rotation. The gluteus medius is also responsible for keeping the pelvis level during walking and running. This lateral hip stabilization is required when you raise a leg to step forward with it. The gluteus medius on the opposite side contracts to keep the weight of the free leg from tilting the pelvis downward on that side. As you walk along, the gluteus medius on either side take turns to support the entire weight of the upper body. They can therefore be overloaded when you carry excess weight while walking.

You can test this lateral stabilization by raising your right leg off the ground. Place your finger on the left side of your hip, just under your iliac crest. You should feel the gluteus medius contracting to dynamically stabilize your pelvis.

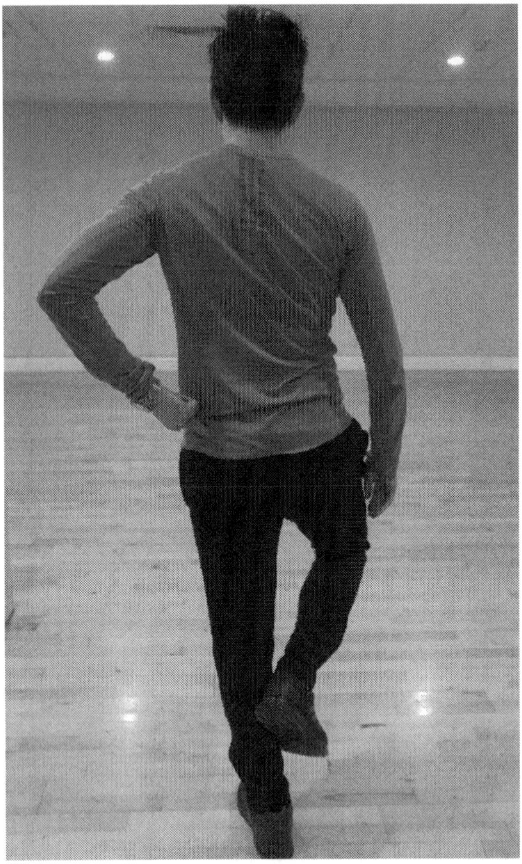

James Tang

Diagram 4.2.6.6: Role of the Gluteus Medius in Lateral Hip Stabilization

All the gluteal muscles have a close relationship. Whilst the maximus, a global muscle composed primarily of type 2 fibres (section 2.3), provides running and jumping power, the medius keeps the hips level during these activities.

Prevention

Avoid standing on one leg to put on your pants or socks, and avoid sitting with cross legs. Avoid prolonged sitting, because this encourages muscle stiffness. Muscles are designed to be moved, and it is detrimental to their health to be held in static positions for a prolonged period. When you sit, your gluteus medius is held in both a shortened and a stretched position;

the anterior part is shortened, and the dorsal part is stretched. Both parts become dysfunctional.

The gluteus medius can contain several active trigger points spaced out evenly across the top portion of the muscle, and they hurt most during walking, slouching in a chair or lying on your back, or when the muscle is directly compressed.

Gluteus medius trigger points are almost always seen in conjunction with quadratus lumborum (QL, section 4.2.6.5) trigger points because these two muscles are strong functional synergists. If a particular activity or posture overloads one of these muscles, it almost always overloads the other one as well. To complicate things further, the referred pain from the QL trigger points can often activate satellite trigger points in the gluteus medius.

Teaching Points

The best way to carry out SMR of the gluteus medius is by using a trigger point ball. You can either lie on the floor with your knees bent at a ninety-degree angle or lean against a wall with the ball placed on the muscle and then roll the ball sideways to search for tender spots. You will often find that the most tender areas are right underneath your iliac crest and the side of your hip, and you need to focus your massage on these areas. As soon as you find a tender area along the muscle, hold on to it until the pain diminishes. Alternatively, you can massage that area and work it with ten to fifteen slow strokes by rolling the ball over this tender area but making sure that you relax and continue to breathe normally throughout the process.

<u>Piriformis</u>

Trigger points are particularly prevalent in the piriformis, and they are a frequent cause of lower back pain. They can develop either through overuse, as in strenuous training and quick changes of direction, or through underuse, as in excessive sitting. Generally, in young people, piriformis tightness is a result of overexertion, especially relating to sports that require a quick change of direction, such as soccer, badminton, and tennis. In old people, it is a result of excessive sitting or prolonged immobility. Tension in the piriformis can put a twist in the sacroiliac joint (chapter 8), adding to your pain.

If you are suffering from active trigger points in the piriformis, especially if you experience the symptoms of piriformis syndrome (section 4.3.2.5), you need to consult a qualified therapist. As with most other muscles that are implicated in lower back pain, piriformis trigger points rarely occur in isolation, and nearly always show up as a component of more complex lower back and hip pain complaints. If you attempt to treat these trigger points in isolation, you are likely to get only short-term results.

Functional Anatomy

The piriformis is one of the hip abductors, but it also eccentrically contracts to decelerate internal rotation and hip adduction (inward rotation of the leg) when the hip is flexed. It is a flat pyramid-shaped muscle of the gluteal region which lies deep under the gluteus maximus. It originates from the anterior surface of the sacrum, and then passes laterally to exit the pelvis through the greater sciatic foramen and inserts onto the greater trochanter of the femur. When the piriformis gets tight, there is a possibility that it can compress the sciatic nerve, leading to sciatica symptoms. When sciatica is caused by a tight piriformis, this is known as piriformis syndrome (section 4.3.2.5). It has been estimated that around 17 per cent of people have a sciatic nerve that runs through the piriformis, making them prone to developing piriformis syndrome when their piriformis is tight, through development of trigger points in it.

Teaching Points

Piriformis trigger points are hidden by the thick gluteus maximus, so penetration must be very focused and deep. You can use a foam roller, but it is far more effective to use a trigger point ball.

Lie face up on the floor with your knees bent at ninety degrees. Roll the ball from the sacrum outwards towards the greater trochanter (i.e., laterally along the buttock), searching for trigger points in the buttocks area deep to the gluteus maximus. Trigger points in this muscle are usually found in the middle of the belly (i.e., midway between the sacrum and the greater trochanter, or between the base of your spine and the front of your hip). Position this spot on top of the trigger point ball and sit firmly down. Keep your back straight and your shoulders up. It is painful to put pressure on a piriformis trigger point, but it is important to maintain deep pressure until the pain dissipates, and then repeat the procedure a couple more times. Again, try to relax and breathe normally.

4.2.7 Cupping Therapy

Cupping therapy is an ancient form of alternative medicine whereby a therapist puts special cups on your skin for a few minutes to create suction. The cups may be made of glass, bamboo, or synthetic materials, such as plastic. This therapy dates back to ancient Egyptian, Chinese, and Middle Eastern cultures. The technique has been in use in China for some three thousand years.

Myofascial cupping is a form of trigger point therapy and myofascial release. This myofascial decompression combines massage and stretching techniques with the use of vacuum cups. Soft tissue is suctioned inside the cups, loosening tissue adhesions (section 4.2.3) by lifting the connective tissues. It also breaks up localized stagnation by enhancing blood and lymphatic circulations so as to improve nutrient supply and drain excess fluids and toxins in stagnant fascia (adhesions) and tight muscle tissues affected by trigger points where circulation has been restricted. Effectively, this is opposite to deep tissue massage, where pressure is applied to tissues. The similarity is that both techniques enhance circulation to the local area, release adhesions, and aid in the removal of accumulated toxins.

A myofascial cupping treatment starts with palpation and massage to locate the target areas. Once these target areas have been located, cups are placed on them and engaged so a negative pressure is created inside. The negative pressure lifts and separates the soft tissue. The longer the cups are kept on, the tighter the suction becomes, but you should avoid keeping the cup on the same spot for more than five minutes. You may use smaller cups to intensify the suction in curvy areas, such as your upper shoulders (when you work on the upper trapezius). Use bigger cups in fleshier areas, such as your back, so they can suck in more of your skin. Blood will then rush to the surface of your skin, causing painless bruises and enabling blood to flow into areas that have been starved of oxygen and nutrients.

An alternative to static suction is gliding. In this process, oil (e.g., grapeseed oil) is rubbed on the skin. Once the cups have been placed on the skin, wait several minutes to maximize the suction effect, and then you can glide the cups over the body. This process pulls fresh oxygen- and nutrient-enriched blood along as the cups move. After several minutes, the cups are removed.

Cupping is usually used as part of a larger series of treatments, and is rarely used as a stand-alone form of therapy. This book explains cupping only as a possible alternative to treating fascial adhesions and trigger points. It neither advocates nor prescribes it as a viable form of therapy. Cupping is generally safe, but you must seek advice and instructions from a qualified professional prior to employing this technique as a self-help treatment for your back pain.

Medical contraindications include those with a tendency to bleed spontaneously, cancer (such as skin tumours or leukaemia), and skin conditions (severe skin allergies or infections). There are other contraindications, and you must therefore seek medical advice first.

You can go online and buy sets of cups in different sizes together with a suction pump, and they are not expensive (diagram 4.2.7). Traditional cups are made of glass, and suction is created by using a tong to hold a burning a piece of cotton wool impregnated with surgical spirit inside the cup. This is held inside the cup momentarily to consume all the oxygen from within it. Then it is immediately inverted and placed over the skin, where the skin is sucked up. Modern cups are made of plastic with a one-way valve at the top and they can be connected to a pump via a plastic tube. You can therefore place the cup wherever it is required and then draw the air out using the pump.

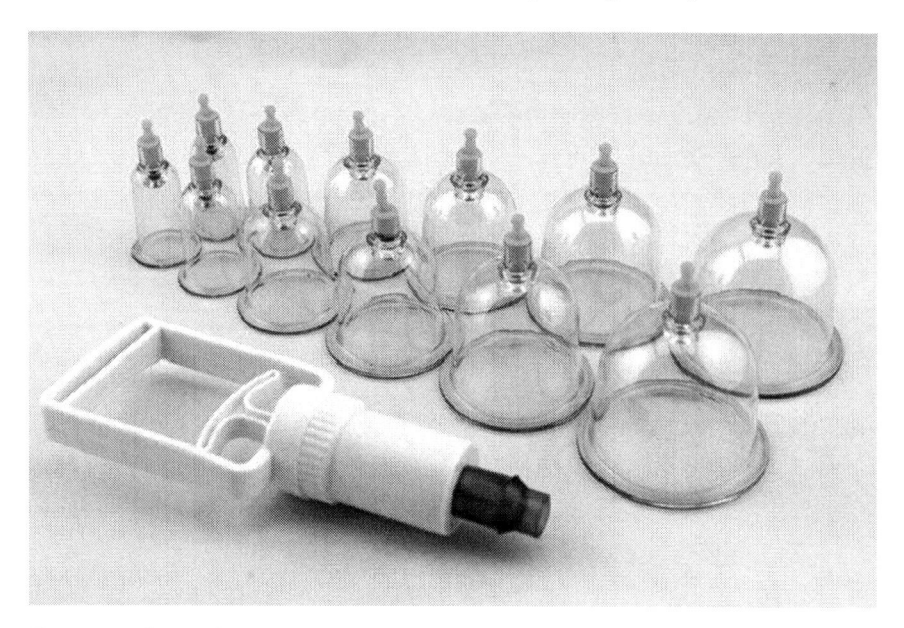

Diagram 4.2.7: Cupping Kit

Conclusion

Please be aware that there are numerous other treatments available for trigger points, such as spray and stretch, dry and wet needling, deep stroking massage, muscle energy and positional release techniques. These are clearly beyond the scope of this book, as they can only be performed by trained professionals and are therefore not considered to be part of the self-management protocol.

You are reminded not to attempt SMR unless you have received explicit guidance from qualified practitioners. After conducting a careful physical examination, your therapist will indicate the location of trigger points that are implicated in your back condition. They will give you guidance as to how to work on them with a view to eradicating them over time. There are many medical contraindications for SMR; these include but are not limited to congestive heart failure, kidney failure (or any organ failure), bleeding disorders, cancer, and contagious skin conditions. If you have any medical issues, you need to seek advice from your doctor prior to undertaking SMR.

Please remember that this is not a textbook on trigger point therapy. It is not the intention of the author to go into great depth on the referral patterns, identification, and treatment of all the possible trigger points that may be implicated in lower back pain. The purpose of this chapter is to:

- Highlight the diversity of symptoms that can be caused by trigger points so you can look out for their involvement as a differential diagnosis in musculoskeletal and other discomforts, such as tendonitis, arthritis, etc.
- Give you an insight into most common muscles that are implicated in lower back pain and how some of their trigger points can be dealt with.

Finally, rest will not solve the problem of myofascial pain, because inactivity is a major perpetuator of trigger points.

4.3 Lengthening Phase

The objective of this phase, following the inhibitory phase of self-myofascial release, is to lengthen the previously tightened muscles by stretching them, thereby improving flexibility.

4.3.1 Introduction to Flexibility

<u>What Is Flexibility?</u>

Being flexible is the ability to move freely through a wide range of movement. Optimal musculoskeletal function requires that an adequate range of motion be maintained in all joints. We should have adequate levels of flexibility, enabling us to take part in a variety of activities. For example, we need to bend our torsos forward to pick things up from the floor or extend our bodies to reach overhead. Flexibility is one of the five components of fitness, the other four being muscular strength, muscular endurance, cardiovascular fitness (stamina), and body composition.

Relevance of Flexibility to Our Modern Lifestyles

Lack of muscular flexibility is prevalent in those who spend a lot of time sitting and maintaining prolonged static postures. As we have already learnt, such postures are detrimental because muscles adapt to the positions we put them in, and the longer we hold them in a certain position, the more tissue adaptation occurs. These adaptations lead to muscle imbalances (section 3.2), predisposing us to musculoskeletal problems, such as neck, knee, shoulder, and back pain. Tight muscles affect the normal range of movement of joints, and of particular importance is the maintenance of muscular flexibility in the lower back and the hamstring regions. Prolonged sitting places the knees in a flexed position precipitating habitual tightness of the hamstrings (section 4.3.2.1). This can cause the hips and pelvis to rotate back, flattening the lower back and causing back problems (section 6.2.7). Tight hamstrings can also be responsible for other back problems, such as sacroiliac joint pain (chapter 8), as they will tend to pull the pelvis out of normal position. Therefore, any exercise routines should include activities that promote muscular flexibility.

Why Do We Need to Be Flexible?

Muscle-strengthening activities develop strength, which helps us to maintain the ability to perform everyday tasks and slows down the rate of osteoporosis and sarcopenia (muscle loss) associated with ageing. But it is imperative that you do not overlook the importance of flexibility.

The benefits of good flexibility include;

- Reduces the likelihood of lower back pain, due to a lack of flexibility in the lower body, particularly in the hamstrings, glutes, and hip flexors.
- Improves postural and muscle imbalances and helps to reduce musculoskeletal pain.
- Increases the range of motion about a joint and increases performance. If your joint is flexible, it requires less energy to move through the range of motion for the exercise you are performing.

- Increases blood flow to the joints.
- Increases coordination, enabling you to perform your daily routines more easily.
- Reduces the risk of injury.

<u>What Limits Our Flexibility?</u>

Factors that affect your flexibility include:

- **Age** – flexibility reduces with age as tissues become less elastic. Accordingly, exercises for the elderly should incorporate flexibility training.

- **Genetics** – some people are more flexible than others, and this may be due to inherited genetics.

- **Gender** – women tend to be more flexible than men.

- **Muscle imbalances** commonly caused by postural dysfunction and prolonged sitting (section 3.2.1).

- **Exercises** – certain activities, where the muscles are not used through their full range of motion, have the potential to reduce flexibility through muscle tightness and adaptive shortening; for example, jogging, football and cycling. Unbalanced resistance training that overdevelops one muscle group (prime movers) while neglecting the opposing muscle group (antagonists) can also cause muscle imbalances that restrict flexibility (section 5.6.4).

- **The strength of the opposing muscle group** – bodybuilders with huge muscle bulks may be strong but they are not as flexible.

- **Joint structure** – while we all have the same general structural foundation, our joints are all shaped a bit differently which can change how flexible we are.

- **Elasticity of the joints, tendons, connective tissue, and muscles**.

How Do We Improve Our Flexibility?

How often do you fail to stretch out your tightened muscles at the end of your workout? The author has observed over the years that the vast majority of gym-goers leave the gym after their workouts without stretching. Stretching helps with the lengthening and increased compliance of your muscle tissues that were made to contract repeatedly during your exercise session. Regular stretching thus enhances your flexibilities with an increased range of motion, but these activities should be performed in a slow, controlled manner with a gradual progression to greater ranges of motion.

It must be emphasized that it is important to warm up (section 5.4.1) for five to ten minutes before stretching.

When Should I Stretch? Should I Stretch Before My Workout?

Stretching before a workout is something we used to do in the olden days, but it has been demonstrated that pre-workout static stretching does not do much to either prepare you for a workout, or reduce your chances of injury. This is because it has been theorized that if you stretch your muscles excessively before your exercise session, it alters the length-tension relationship (section 2.6) of the muscles that you stretch, reducing the contractile force of those muscles and hence affecting your performance. This is the rationale of performing pre-workout dynamic stretches (section 5.6.1) and post-workout static stretches.

4.3.2 Practical Advice on Stretches

Muscles that are typically shortened are the postural muscles. Examples of these include the following:

- Hamstrings (section 4.3.2.1)
- Hip flexors (e.g. Psoas major) (section 4.3.2.2)
- Adductors (section 4.3.2.3)
- Tensor fasciae latae (TFL) (section 4.3.2.4)
- Piriformis (section 4.3.2.5)

- Quadratus lumborum (section 4.3.2.6)
- Erector spinae (section 4.3.2.7)
- Rectus femoris (section 4.3.2.8)

The Best Way to Stretch

There are numerous types of stretch which may accomplish different objectives. For example, there is PNF (**proprioceptive neuromuscular facilitation**—often carried out by an experienced therapist), as well as ballistic, static and dynamic stretches (Section 5.6.1), but we will only focus on static stretches in this section.

Static stretches can either be active or passive. If a partner or another group of muscles assists in the stretching process, it is known as an active stretch. This can be achieved by contraction of the agonist to stretch the antagonist group of muscles. A typical example of this involves contraction of the tiberalis anterior (the largest muscle located in the anterior [front] compartment of your leg) to stretch the calf.

There are two types of static passive stretches: maintenance and developmental. We will use the static stretch of your hamstrings as an example.

4.3.2.1 Hamstring Stretch

Functional Anatomy

Hamstrings are a group of three muscles located at the back of your thigh: bicep femoris, semitendinosus muscle, and semimembranosus muscle. Each hamstring originates from the ischial tuberosity of the pelvis, crosses the hip and the knee joints, and attaches to the tibia or fibula. This means that when they contract, they can either extend your hips (i.e., move your legs backwards so they are synergists of the gluteus maximus in hip extension) or flex (bend) your knees. Whilst the hamstrings are able to produce both movements simultaneously, they cannot do so to their full capacity. It is one movement or the other if you are looking to go all the way with a hamstring contraction.

Tight hamstrings can cause the pelvis to rotate back (resulting in posterior pelvic tilt), flattening the lower back by reducing your natural lordotic curve. In fact, tight hamstrings play a major role in flat back posture (section 6.2.7). This postural deviation is disadvantageous for the spine, as it causes imbalances to the muscles that are attached to the lumbo-pelvic-hip complex, as well as predisposing you to disc injury, due to the constant pulling of the shortened muscles increasing pressure on the vertebrae. Tight hamstrings can also play a role in sacroiliac dysfunction (chapter 8).

An example of a static maintenance stretch for the hamstrings:

Teaching Points (Diagram 4.3.2.1)

Lie on your back and raise one leg off the floor. Keeping your leg straight, place both hands behind it and pull it in slightly closer to your chest until you feel a little tension. Hold this position until the tension subsides, and then relax. Do this three to four times.

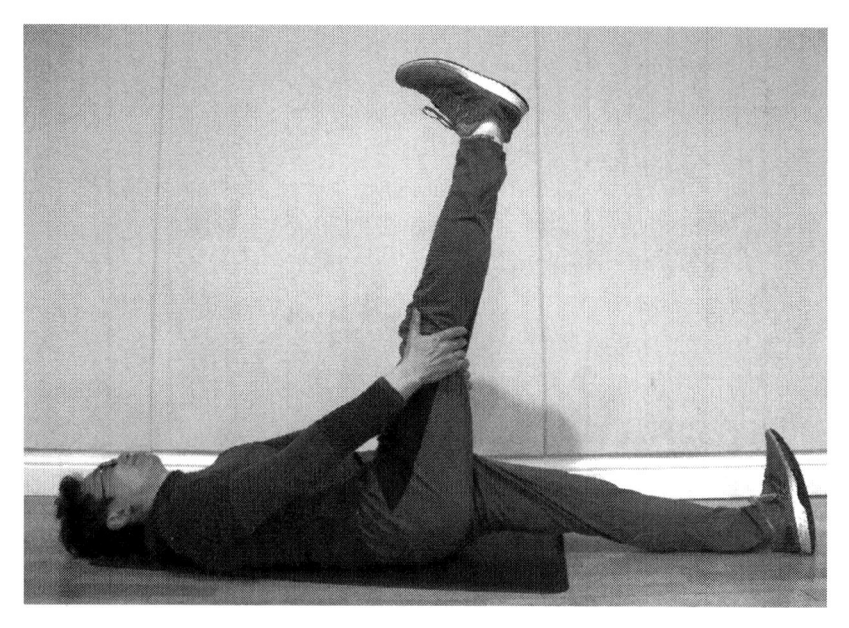

Diagram 4.3.2.1: Hamstring Stretch

An example of a static developmental stretch for the hamstrings:

If you are unable to touch your toes when you flex your hips, your hamstrings (and possibly your glutes as well) are probably too tight. Static developmental stretches can help to lengthen your hamstrings and significantly improve your flexibility over time.

The procedure is similar to that of the maintenance stretch mentioned above, but when the initial tension subsides, instead of relaxing and waiting for the next stretch, take the stretch further. When the tension again subsides, take it further one more time.

4.3.2.2 Hip Flexor Stretch

Let us take a look at the anatomy of this very important culprit in hyperlordosis (section 6.2.1) and lower back pain. There are basically three hip flexor muscles:

- **Psoas major**: This muscle originates from transverse processes T12–L5.
- **Iliacus**: This muscle originates from the iliac fossa and inserts to the lesser trochanter of the femur.
- **Rectus femoris**: Part of the quadriceps group of muscles, the rectus femoris originates from the anterior inferior iliac spine and attaches to the tibia via the common patella tendon.

The most important hip flexor is the psoas major, together with the iliacus, often referred to as the **iliopsoas**. The role of the hip flexors is to flex your hip.

Prolonged sitting causes your hips to stay in a flexed position, shortening your hip flexors. When these muscles are tight, not only do they "turn off" their antagonists (section 3.5), the glute muscles, but they also pull the pelvis forward, leading to an anterior tilting of the pelvis, which leads to imbalances of the muscles that are attached to the lumbo-pelvic-hip complex. (Please refer to section 6.2.1 for hyperlordosis).

Teaching Points (Diagram 4.3.2.2)

You should focus on stretching the psoas major and not the rectus femoris. You must therefore stay tall, keeping your torso upright throughout the stretch, and resist the temptation to lean forward into the stretch. You can stretch the hip flexors more effectively by contracting your glutes, as this will "switch off", or relax, the hip flexors through reciprocal inhibition (section 3.5). However, you may not yet be able to activate your glutes at this stage (section 4.4.2.1) while performing this stretch, although it is beneficial to do so.

- Kneel with one knee on the floor and the other foot in front with the knee bent.
- Push your hips forward and keep the back upright.
- Stretch to mild tension and hold for as long as it takes until you feel the tension diminishing.
- Switch legs to get a balanced stretch.

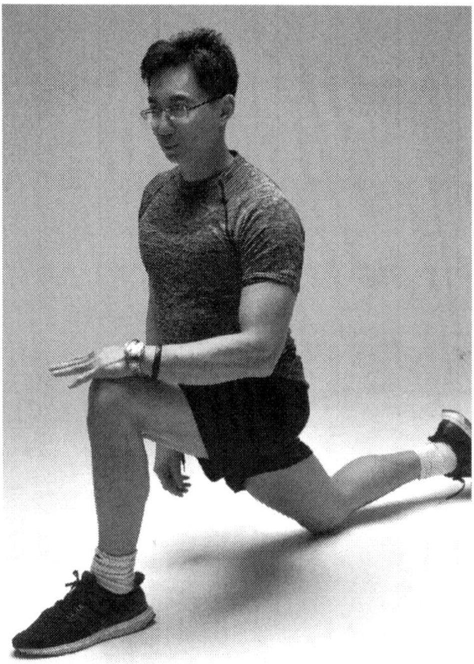

Diagram 4.3.2.2: Hip Flexor Stretch

4.3.2.3 Adductor Stretches

<u>Functional Anatomy</u>

These are the inside leg muscles, commonly referred to as the groin. The main action of these muscles is to pull the leg inward. They are very important in sports such as soccer where the adductors are used in kicking a ball with the inside of the foot. They are also used in flexion and extension of the thigh when running, or moving against resistance.

There are five adductor muscles: the pectineus, the gracilis, the adductor longus, the brevis, and the magnus.

The adductors work in opposition to the abductors, which are located on the outside of the hip. Together, they play an important role in pelvic positioning, which in turn can affect your spinal alignment. As a result, one way to positively influence the flexibility of your lower back is to release both the inner and outer thigh muscles.

<u>Seated Adductor Stretch 1 (Diagrams 4.2.2.3)</u>

Teaching Points

Sit on the floor, place the soles of your feet together, and let your knees drop out to the sides. If your adductors are very tight, your knees will not go down very far. You should feel a good stretch in your groin. Stay in this position until you feel the tension releasing. Repeat between three and five times.

<u>Seated Adductor Stretch 2</u>

Teaching Points

Sit on the floor but extend your legs out to the sides, making as wide a *V* shape as you comfortably can.

To progress, pivot forward from your hip towards the floor. Again, go only as far as you can without pain or discomfort. The torso needs to be kept straight at all times, and there should be no curving of your upper back. Maintain the position for about five to ten seconds, and breathe normally.

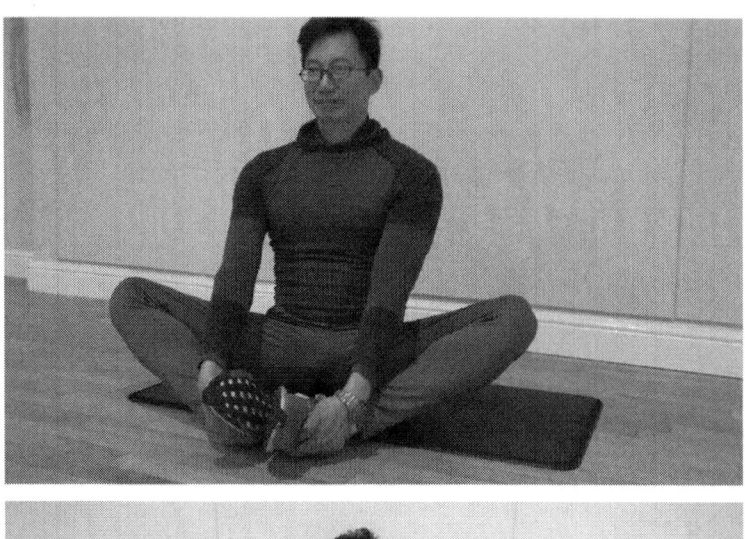

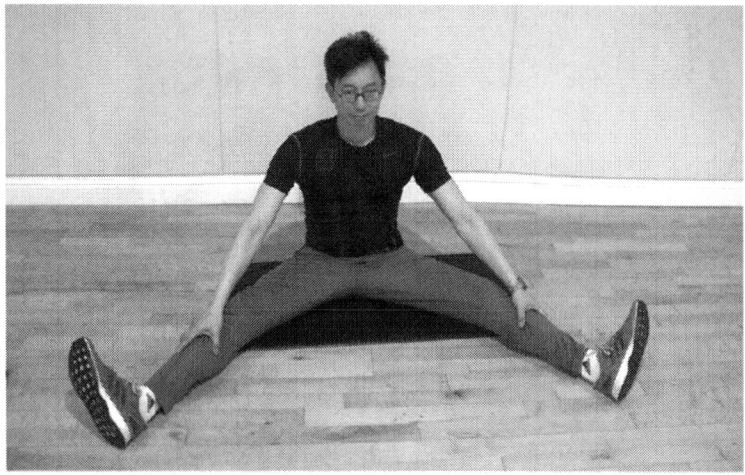

Diagrams 4.3.2.3: Seated Adductor Stretches

4.3.2.4 Tensor Fasciae Latae (TFL) and Iliotibial Band (IT Band) Stretch

Functional Anatomy

The TFL muscle, one of the four abductors, originates from the upper anterior portion of the pelvis, and inserts into the iliotibial band (ITB). The ITB is a tendinous structure extending from the gluteus maximus and the TFL. The ITB inserts at the fibular head, the lateral patellar retinaculum, and Gerdy's tubercle on the lateral aspect of the tibia.

The ITB is designed to assist the hip muscles in abduction of the thigh and to stabilize the side of the knee. Since the ITB is not a very strong structure, weakness in surrounding muscles and overuse can lead to injury. Typically, when the gluteus medius is weakened due to reciprocal inhibition (section 3.5) by the hip flexors as a result of prolonged sitting, the TFL (synergist of the gluteus medius in hip abduction) will become synergistically dominant (Section 3.6), and because it is attached through the ITB down to the lateral side of the leg to the knee, it can cause an excessive lateral pull on the patella, resulting in it rubbing against the outside of the thigh bone, and misalignment of the patella, and finally, lateral knee pain.

This irritation to the ITB is known as **ITB syndrome**. It has been a source of pain for those who overtrain or who train incorrectly, and is one of the most common overuse injuries in runners and cyclists. ITB syndrome is the inflammation of the ITB as it rubs against the outside of the knee joint. Symptoms include pain over the outside of the knee which will come on gradually over time, getting progressively worse until running must stop; sometimes, ITB syndrome is accompanied by a clicking sensation, which is a result of the ITB tightening and snapping across the joint during activity.

Treatment programmes include stretching the ITB, and the following set of stretches will address both the TFL and the ITB band.

Teaching Points (Diagram 4.3.2.4)

Stand adjacent to a wall, using the arm closest to the wall to provide support. The leg closest to the wall is crossed behind the opposite leg. To create the stretch, bend the torso away from the wall. To get more stretch, you can bring your hands together above your head. Bend away from the wall while keeping your arms extended overhead. Repeat on the other side.

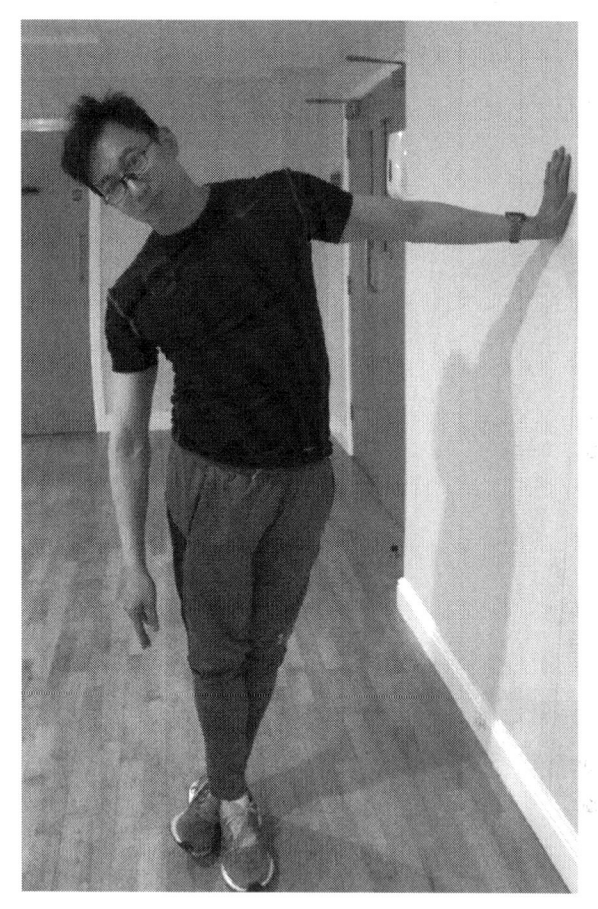

Diagram 4.3.2.4: TFL Stretch

4.3.2.5 Piriformis Stretch

The piriformis is a very important gluteal muscle, and it is prone to being tight. Generally speaking, in young people, piriformis tightness results from overexertion. In old people, it results from excessive sitting or prolonged immobility. Prolonged sitting leads to weakness of the glutes via reciprocal inhibition through tightness of the hip flexors. The glutes are responsible for hip extension (backward movement of your legs), and if the glutes are not performing their task properly, the piriformis (amongst other synergist muscles) has to pick up the slack. Because they have to work harder and more often, they become chronically tight. This is a typical example of synergistic dominance (section 3.6). Here, the synergist (the piriformis) is taking over the role of the prime mover.

Functional Anatomy (Please refer to Section 4.2.6.6)

Sciatica is a symptom and not a disease on its own, and it occurs when pressure is put directly on the sciatic nerve in some way. The principal presenting symptom is shooting pain in the buttock and down the back of the leg. However, the symptoms can vary widely from mild tingling, dull ache or burning sensation to, in some cases, severe pain that can cause immobility. The pain may get worse at night or after standing or sitting for a long period of time. Sciatica pain usually goes away within six weeks unless there are serious underlying conditions. Sciatica is often associated with back pain, but it can happen independently.

The sciatic nerve is the largest and longest single nerve in the human body. It is about as big as your thumb at its widest point. It originates in the lower spine, where nerve roots exit the spinal cord, and it extends all the way down the back of the leg to the toes.

Piriformis syndrome is a condition in which sciatica pain is caused by the piriformis being tight. This occurs because the sciatic nerve is close to the piriformis (the sciatic nerve emerges from the sciatic foramen inferiorly to the piriformis). However, most cases of sciatica are not due to piriformis syndrome, but as a result of herniation of the intervertebral disc pressing on the roots of the sciatic nerve in the lower back.

Teaching Points (Diagram 4.3.2.5)

Lie on your back with both knees bent at ninety degrees. The ankle associated with the piriformis muscle to be stretched should be placed on the front of your other knee. Using your hands, pull the thigh of this leg in towards your chest. Hold this position for twenty to thirty seconds, or until the tension decreases. Then take the stretch further until the tension subsides once again.

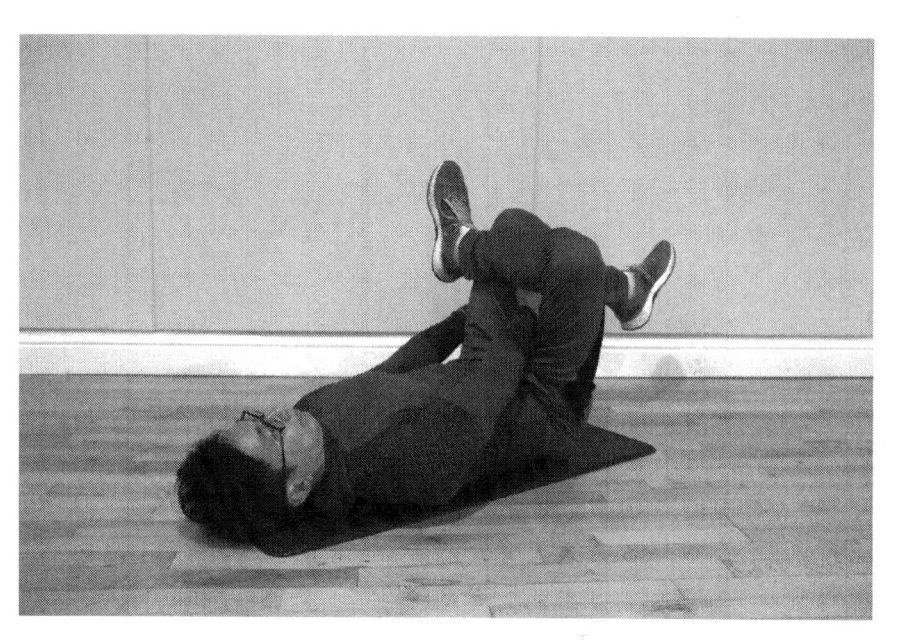

Diagram 4.3.2.5: Piriformis Stretch

4.3.2.6 Quadratus Lumborum (QL) Stretch

<u>Functional Anatomy (please refer to section 4.2.6.5)</u>

There are a number of QL stretches that can be used to help prevent lower back pain. One example is the simple side stretch demonstrated below (Diagram 4.3.2.6a).

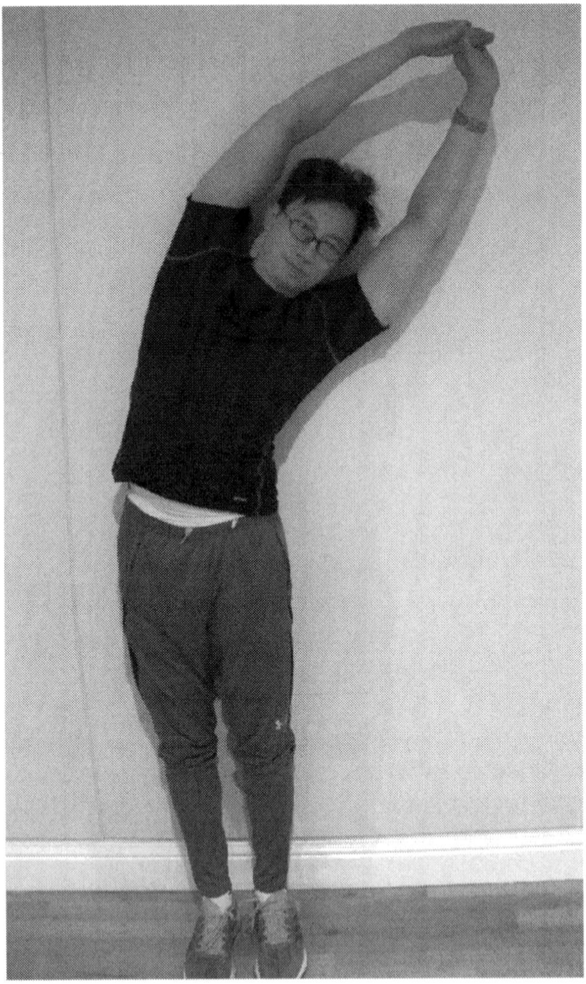

Diagram 4.3.2.6a: QL Standing Side Stretch

Alternatively, you can challenge your core stability by lying sideways and stretching the QL on a Swiss stability ball (Diagram 4.3.2.6b).

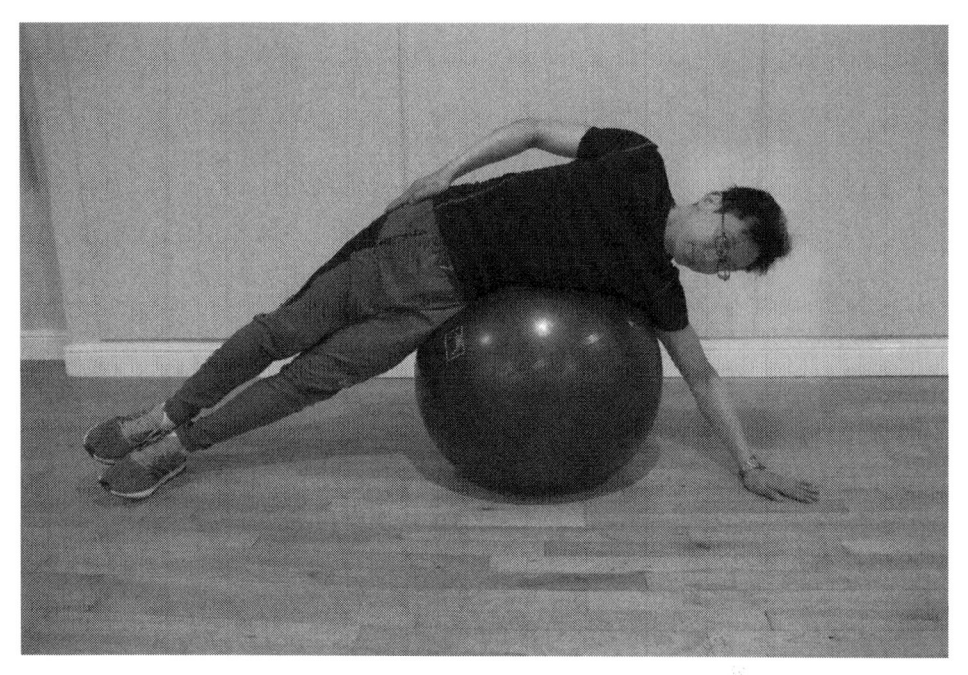

Diagram 4.3.2.6b:—QL Side Stretch on a Stability Ball

Please remember that these are only examples of stretches for the QL; there are plenty of other alternatives available. Please speak to your therapist or exercise professional, who will give you guidance on the most suitable QL stretch for you.

4.3.2.7 Erector Spinae Stretch

Tightness of the erector spinae is prevalent in those with hyperlordotic (section 6.2.1) and swayback (section 6.2.4) postures, which can be caused by excessive abdominal obesity. Stretching the erector spinae is therefore part of the corrective exercise protocol for hyperlordosis (section 6.3).

Besides hyperlordosis, these muscles can also be strained due to improper lifting techniques and frequent bending. If your lower back feels stiff, this muscle may be the culprit. It is important to stretch it out if you want to keep your lower back moving and feeling good.

Functional Anatomy (please refer to section 4.2.6.4)

Teaching Points (Diagram 4.3.2.7)

All three of these muscles can be stretched simultaneously because they all perform the same actions. Since these muscles extend the spine, you need to flex (bend forward) your spine to stretch them. It is important to perform these stretches gently, since it can be dangerous to aggressively flex your spine.

Kneeling Stretches

With your buttocks resting back on your heels and your arms reaching out in front of you, stretch the erector spinae, which runs from the back of your pelvis up along the bones of your spine in your lower back. It is advisable to stretch your lumbar erector spinae daily. Hold the stretch for at least thirty seconds and perform three or more repetitions.

Forward Bends

Stand with your feet hip-width apart. Bend forward, pivoting from your hips. If your lower back, glutes, or hamstrings are tight, your back may be rounded (as demonstrated in diagram 4.3.2.7) and you may not be able to touch your toes with your fingers. Just hold your elbows and let your head hang down. Hold this stretch for about thirty seconds. Inhale when you come up slowly using the strength of your legs, and not your lower back.

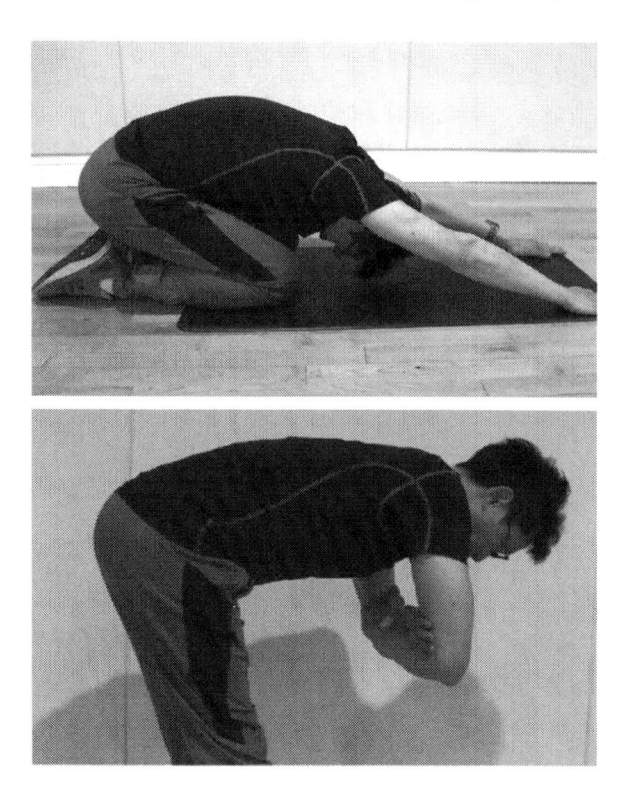

A Practical Guide to the Self-Management of Lower Back Pain

Diagram 4.3.2.7: Erector Spinae—Kneeling Stretch and Forward Bend

4.3.2.8 Rectus Femoris Stretch

This is one of the four quadriceps muscles. The main function of the quadriceps is to extend your knees. The rectus femoris, along with the iliopsoas, is one of the hip flexor muscles (section 4.3.2.2), and is responsible for moving the legs forward when you walk or run. If the rectus femoris is tight, it can inhibit the glutes (section 3.5) and limit hip extension, subsequently shortening stride length. It can also pull the pelvis forward, causing an anterior pelvic tilt, which in turn tightens the hamstrings and can predispose you to lower back pain (see section 6.2.1 on hyperlordosis).

Anatomy

The four quadriceps muscles are the vastus lateralis, vastus medialis, vastus intermedius, and rectus femoris. All the quadriceps muscles attach to the patella (kneecap). Each of the vastus muscles originates on the femur and they are partially covered by the rectus femoris. Unlike the vastus muscles, the rectus femoris originates from the anterior inferior iliac spine (AIIS) of your hip, making it also a hip flexor muscle.

Teaching Points (Diagram 4.3.2.8)

This stretch combines the actions of knee flexion and hip extension. Stand facing a wall and rest your left hand on the wall for support. Grasp the toes of your right foot with your right hand and gently pull the foot towards your right buttock. Keep your inner thighs together, and your back upright. Increase the stretch by slowly moving your right knee back. Hold the position for up to thirty seconds or as long as it takes for the tension to dissipate. Relax briefly and repeat up to four times. Repeat the same stretch on your left leg.

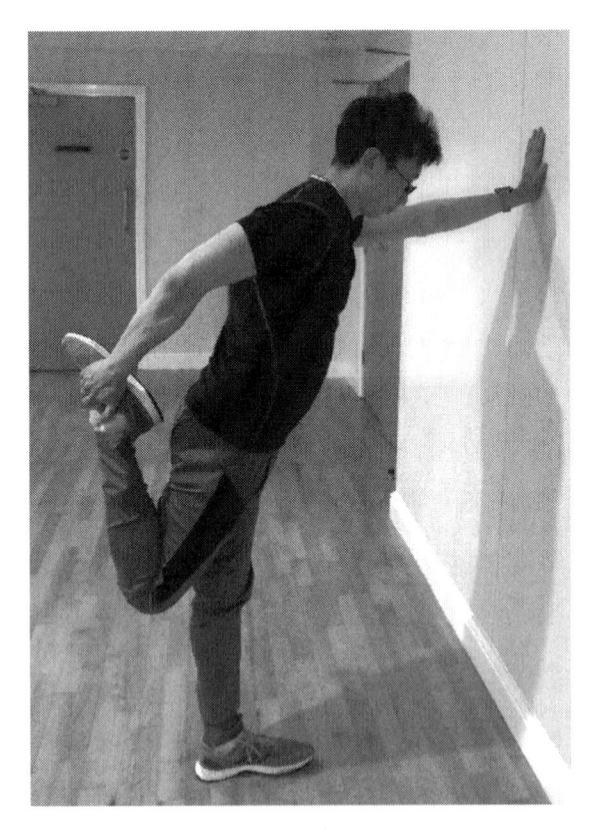

Diagram 4.3.2.8: Rectus Femoris Stretch

A Word of Caution

If you have a degenerative spine condition, injury or ongoing back or neck pain, consult your physician before embarking on a new fitness routine. Always proceed with caution and listen to your body's cues; sharp, painful sensations indicate that you have stretched too far. It is important to always warm up before stretching (section 5.4.1). Never bounce when stretching, as this can tear muscle.

You may be interested in other activities that are good for flexibility, including yoga, tai chi, and Pilates. The author would recommend that you try Iyengar yoga, a type of yoga that enhances your core strength, balance, and flexibility.

Only a limited number of stretches for the most common muscle groups implicated in lower back pain have been mentioned in this chapter. There could be other muscles involved in your lower back condition, and there are plenty of alternative stretches and techniques available. The hold time and repetitions for the various stretches mentioned in this chapter are for general guidance only. Please consult your therapist and exercise professional for the type of flexibility training that is appropriate for your own individual requirements.

4.4 Activation Phase

4.4.1 Introduction to Activation

You need to activate those muscles that are typically weakened, including:

- Gluteus maximus and medius (section 4.4.2.1)
- Quadratus lumborum (QL) (section 4.4.2.2)
- Transversus abdominis (section 4.4.2.3)
- Multifidis
- Middle/lower trapezius and the rhomboids, which are typically related to hyperkyphosis (section 6.4).

You need to perform these activities regularly, because the more you practise them, the more efficient your brain becomes in instructing these muscles to work, resulting in the enhancement of your neuromuscular efficiency.

4.4.2 Practical Advice on Activation

4.4.2.1 Activation of Gluteal Muscles

<u>Activation of the Gluteus Maximus</u>

Functional Anatomy (please refer to section 4.2.6.6)

The gluteus maximus, gluteus medius, and gluteus minimus are collectively referred to as the glutes or the gluteal muscles. They are the key stabilizer muscles around the hip joint.

Sitting for a prolonged period causes your hip flexors to be tight, and as a result of reciprocal inhibition (section 3.5), your glutes can become inhibited and weakened.

Teaching Points

The glute bridge (see diagram 4.4.2.1a below) is probably one of the most useful glute activation exercises, but its benefit is often negated by poor technique.

Lie on the floor on your back. Bend your knees at a ninety-degree angle, and place your feet flat on the floor. Contract or squeeze your glutes (you should be able to feel them tightening) to lift your hips and thighs off the floor, keeping your back straight at all times. Maintain a neutral spine, and tighten your core. It is important that you use neither your lower back nor your hamstrings to perform this exercise.

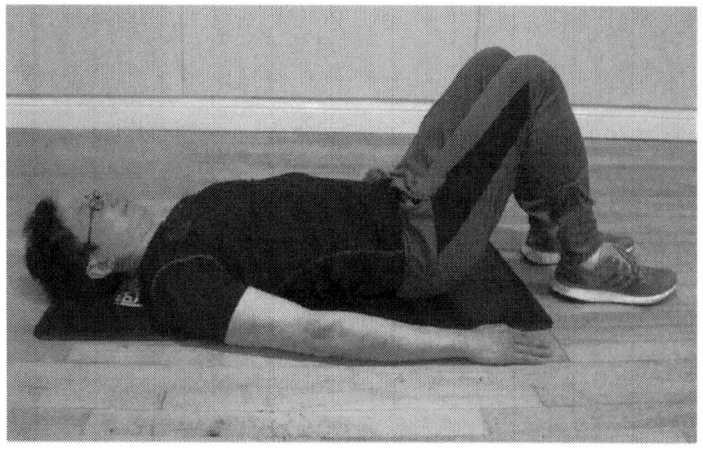

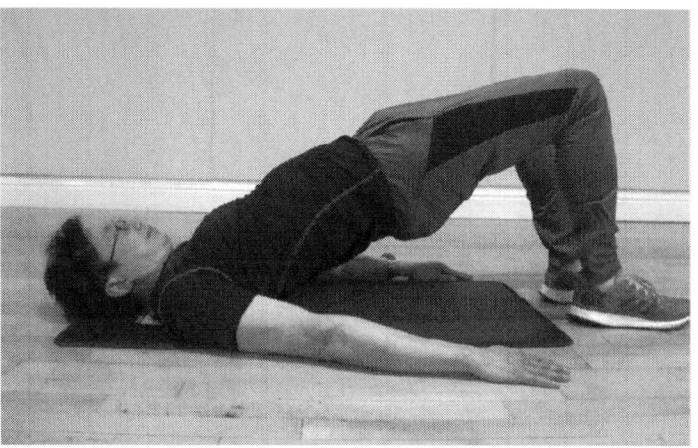

Diagram 4.4.2.1a: Glute Bridge

Progressions

When you can manage the standard glute bridge with confidence, you can bridge with just one leg (see diagram 4.4.2.1b), or you can even challenge your core stability by using a Swiss ball or TRX cable.

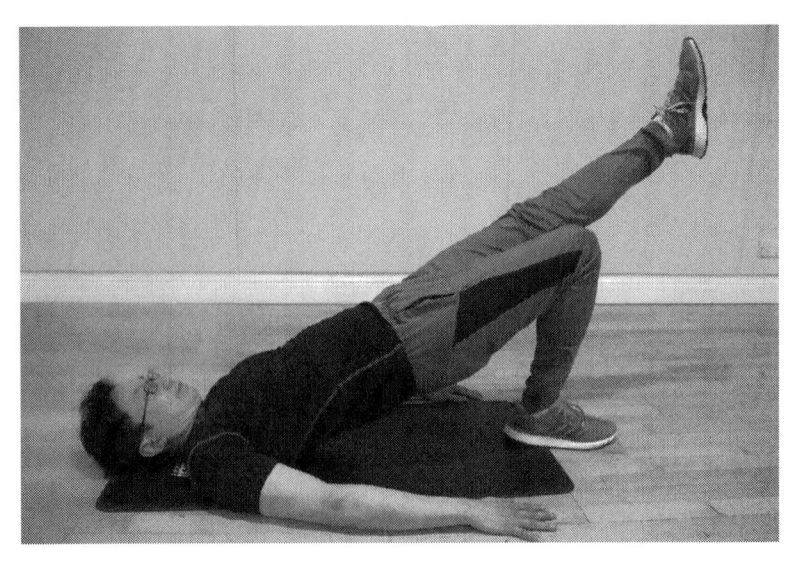

Diagram 4.4.2.1b: Single-Leg Glute Bridge

Other Glute Activation Exercises

- Cable standing hip extension (Diagram 4.4.2.1c)
- Dead lifts
- Squats (with or without weight)
- Body weight squats
- Lunges (with or without weight).

Please remember that these are only a small selection of activations and strengthening exercises for your glutes. It is important to realize that everyone is different. It must be again emphasized that it is important to engage an exercise professional who can devise activities to suit your own individual requirements. For instance, if you have hypertension, performing the glute bridge in a supine position may be contraindicated; you may be better off doing an isolated glute activation exercise using a cable machine (diagram 4.4.2.1c). The same applies for those with knee problems.

Teaching points:

- Hook an ankle cuff to a low cable pulley and then attach the cuff to your ankle.

- Face the weight stack from a distance of approximately two feet, grasping the frame for support. Do not swing your hips from side to side during the exercise. You should only be extending your working leg back.

- Keep your knees and hips slightly bent with your core engaged. Consciously contract your glutes to slowly extend the working leg back in a semicircular arc. At the top, squeeze your glutes momentarily before flexing your working leg forward until you reach the starting position.

- Follow the recommended number of repetitions advised by your trainer, and then switch legs and repeat.

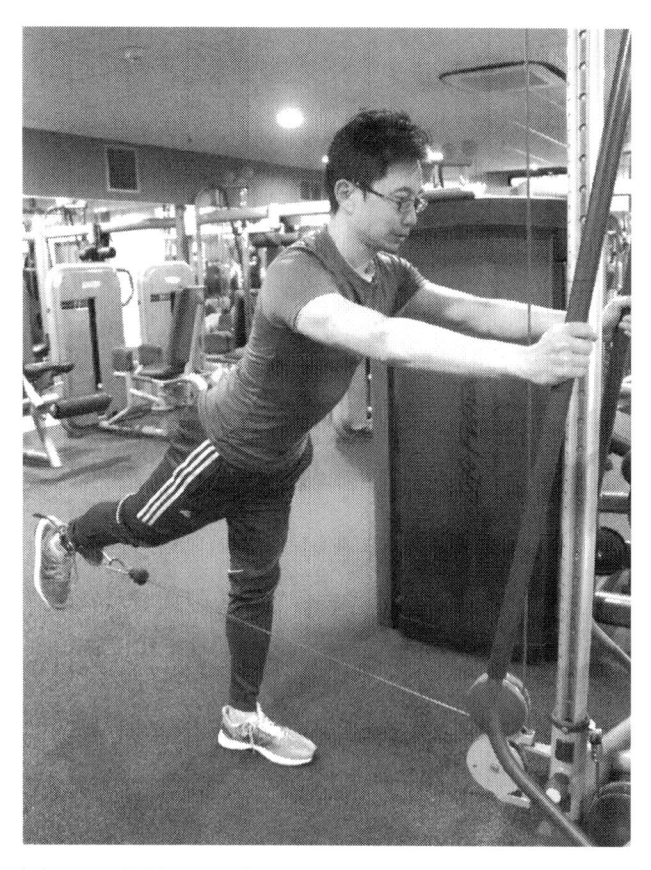

Diagram 4.4.2.1c: Cable Standing Hip Extension

Activation of the Gluteus Medius

Functional Anatomy (please refer to section 4.2.6.6)

The gluteus medius also gets "turned off" due to prolonged sitting, and weakness of this muscle will not only predispose you to lower back pain, but also knee pain. This is because if the gluteus medius is weak, the tensor fasciae latae (TFL) muscle (section 4.3.2.4) will become synergistically dominant, and because it is attached through the iliotibial band (ITB) down the lateral side of the leg to the knee, it can cause excessive lateral pull on the patella, resulting in misalignment and finally lateral knee pain. So if you have lateral knee pain, it may not be due to arthritis; it could simply be due to tightness of the TFL, resulting from a weak gluteus medius.

Exercises that you can do for activation of the gluteus medius include side-lying hip abduction (see *diagram 4.4.2.1d*), seated hip abduction, and standing cable hip abduction.

Teaching Points for Side-Lying Hip Raise (Diagram 4.4.2.1d)

- Lie on your side, keep both knees bent, and flex the hips to about thirty degrees.
- While keeping your heels touching and your pelvis stationary, separate your knees by contracting your gluteus medius. Perform this action slowly and under control.
- You can place your hand on your gluteus medius (just below your iliac crest under your lower back) to ensure that it is contracting whilst performing the exercise.
- Perform fifteen repetitions and switch sides.

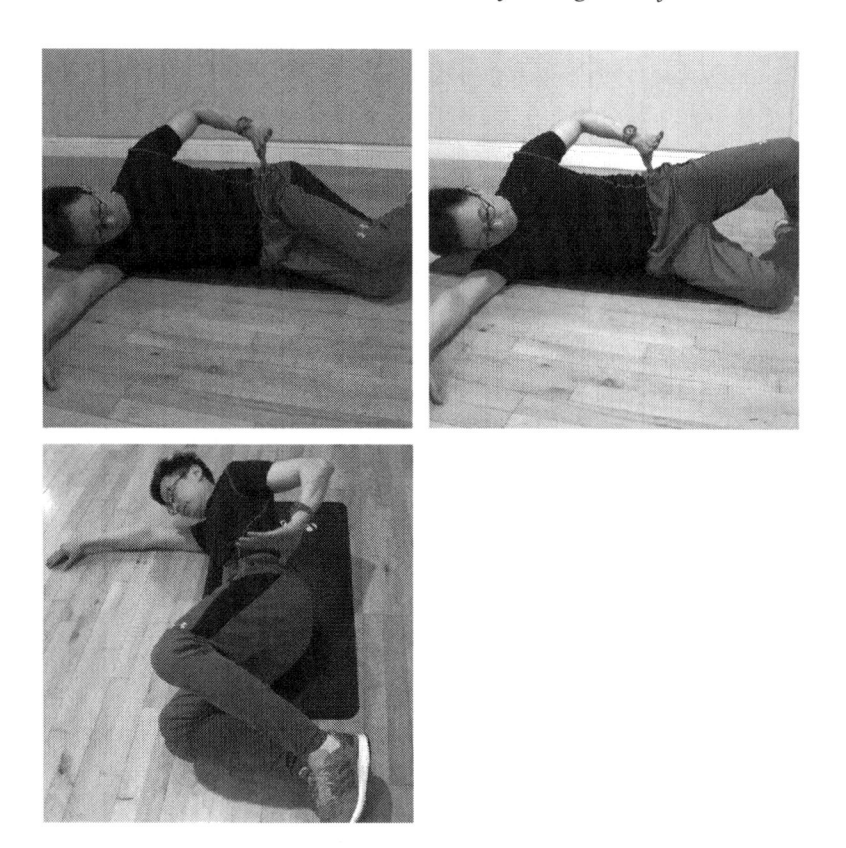

Diagram 4.4.2.1d: Side-Lying Hip Abduction

To progress, you can perform the same exercise but abduct with straight rather than bent legs.

4.4.2.2 Activation of the Quadratus Lumborum (QL)

A simple way to test the strength of your QL is to check how long you can hold a side plank (section 4.4.3). If you are able to hold it for one minute on one side but only thirty seconds on the other, you have muscle imbalances between your left and right QLs. In this case, you will need to strengthen and place more emphasis on the weaker side.

Weakened QL muscles can lead to recurring lower back pain. Keeping your QL strong will also help you to improve the way you perform everyday actions, such as bending from your waist. Exercises for strengthening the

QL include side bends on a stability ball, as well as side planks. The side plank is an isometric core-strengthening exercise that targets your QL as well as your internal and external oblique muscles.

4.4.2.3 Activation of the Transversus Abdominis (TvA)

<u>Functional Anatomy</u>

The TvA originates from the iliac crest, inguinal ligament, thoracolumbar fascia, and the lower six ribs, and it inserts into the xiphoid process of the sternum, linea alba, and pubic crest. This is a very important, if not the most important, muscle of the core; its main role is to stabilize the lower back and pelvis before movement of the limbs.

You are reminded that the core muscles consist of the diaphragm at the top, pelvic floor muscles at the base of the abdominal cavity, and the multifidus muscles posteriorly (section 3.3.2.2). The TvA wraps around your torso, functioning like a corset. It is these muscles, working together, that make it possible to move efficiently and transfer power to the arms and legs. Core dysfunction is a common cause of lower back pain (section 3.3).

<u>Activation of the TvA (Core Activation)</u>

The TVA and the other core musculatures become weak as a result of prolonged sitting. These core muscles are not used when one is constantly sitting in a stable environment, and they are neurologically turned off over time.

To feel the TvA contracting, try to stand up and place your finger on the bony prominence at the side of your hip (your anterior superior iliac spine). Run your finger towards the centre, and then cough. You should be able to feel the TVA contracting.

<u>Teaching Points</u>

Lie on your back with your knees bent at ninety degrees. Exhale, contract your abdomen, and pull your belly button towards your spine and tilt your pelvis up very slightly. (One of the functions of the TvA is to create a posterior pelvic tilt, thus negating the effect of the anterior pelvic tilt.) You should be able to feel the muscle contracting if you press two inches in from the bony prominence at the front of your pelvis. Breathe normally whilst maintaining an isometric hold of this position for six to ten seconds. Release and repeat for three sets of fifteen repetitions.

It must be emphasized that it is not enough just to know how to activate your core; you need to consciously maintain activation of your TvA during all functional activities, including whenever you are walking, running, and most importantly, performing your workouts (**abdominal bracing**).

4.4.3 Core-Strengthening Exercises

Once you have learnt how to consciously activate your TVA, you need to progress to enhance its isometric strength (section 5.6.7) so as to keep your core and other abdominal muscles strong and stable. Core-strengthening exercises should therefore be an integral part of any workout programme, because a strong core helps to stabilize, balance, and power the body during any functional activities. In fact, core strength is the basis for all coordinated and powerful functional movements.

Please note that the exercises listed below are only examples and that this is not an exhaustive list of core-strengthening activities. You need to consult your exercise professional for the most appropriate core-strengthening programme for you. They will also be able to monitor your form, and offer you progression to further challenge your body.

<u>The Plank</u>

For most people, the primary goal of performing the plank exercise is not to burn calories, but to strengthen the muscles of the core because the plank is an isometric exercise as it does not involve any movement. That said, doing any exercise that engages more muscles will inevitably increase your calorie consumption, and the plank exercise below is no exception.

You can progress to this basic core-strengthening exercise once you have mastered the conscious activation of your TvA (section 4.4.2.3). You must

James Tang

keep your TvA activated (maintain isometric contraction of the TvA) throughout your plank exercise.

Teaching Points (Diagram 4.4.3a)

- Begin in the plank position with your forearms and toes on the floor.

- Keep your torso straight (i.e., keep your body in a straight line from head to toes with no sagging or bending). A lot of people either elevate their bottom (see bottom picture of diagram 4.4.3a) or hyperextend their spine (see diagram 4.4.3b) during this exercise. In these incorrect positions, there is compression of the spinal discs at some point in the spine, and this will increase the risk of spinal disc injury over time.

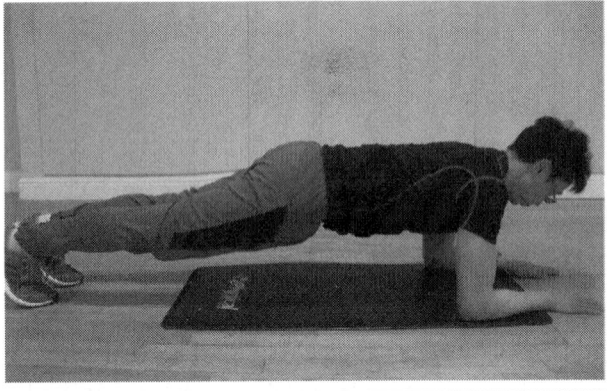

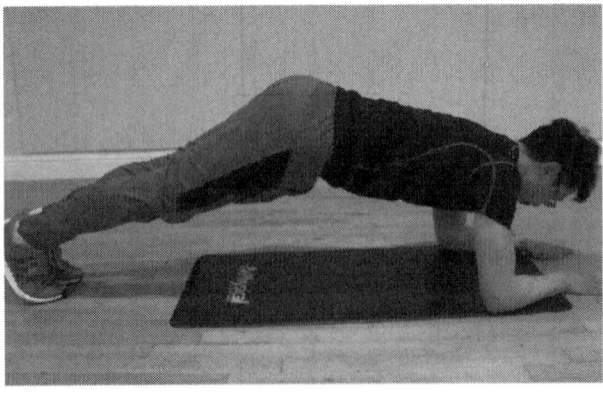

Diagram 4.4.3a: The Plank

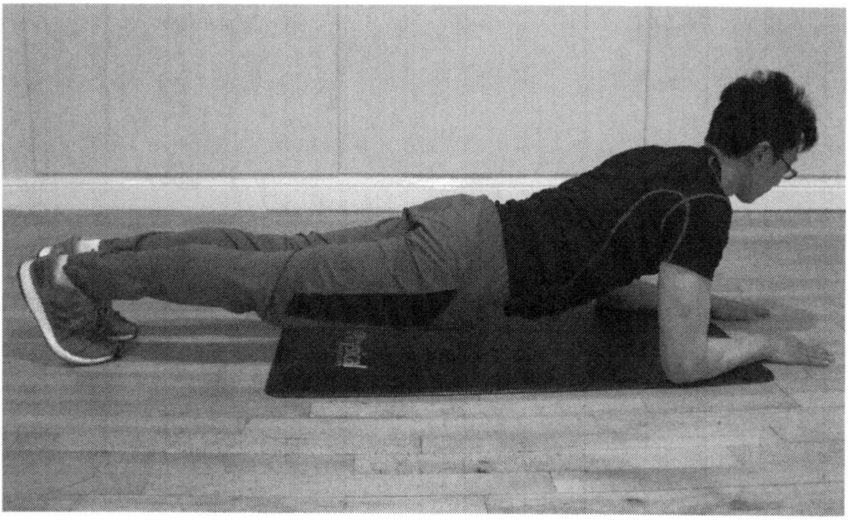

Diagram 4.4.3b: The Plank with Excessive Spinal Extension

- Keep your head relaxed; you should be looking at the floor.
- Hold this position for as long as you can, keeping the TvA activated while breathing normally. Starts with thirty seconds, and then progress to one or two minutes, and so on.

Progression of the Basic Plank

Plank with Leg Lift

Teaching Points

Adopt the same plank position as mentioned above, with your forearms and toes on the floor. Then, slowly raise one leg off the floor. Hold momentarily, and slowly lower your leg to the floor. Then, switch legs and repeat. Perform three to four sets of at least twelve repetitions. These are endurance exercises for type 1 fibres (section 2.3), and the repetition range should be in excess of twelve (section 5.6.2).

James Tang

Plank with Leg Raise and Arm Lift (Diagram 4.4.3c)

Teaching Points

Begin from the same plank position as above. Carefully shift your weight to your right forearm and extend your left arm straight out in front of you. Hold momentarily, but remember to engage your TvA throughout the exercise and breathe normally. Then, slowly bring your arm back to the starting position. Switch arms and repeat. Perform three to four sets of at least twelve reps.

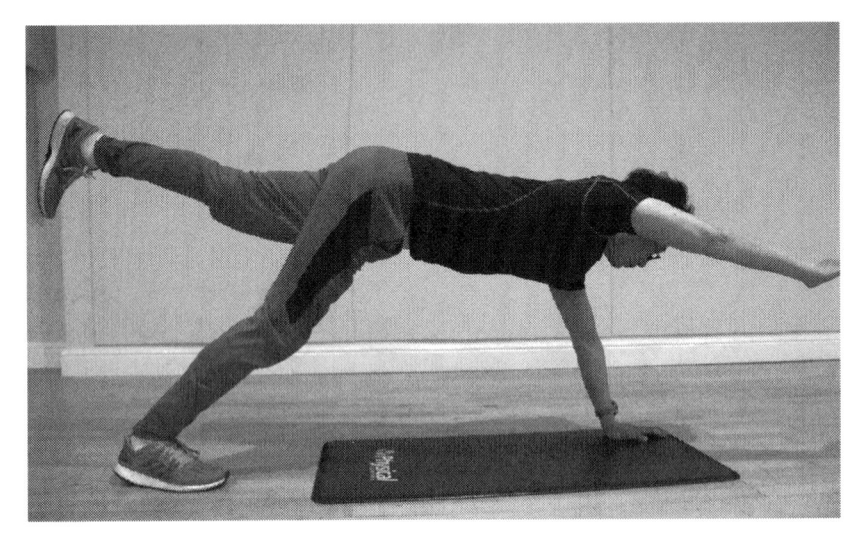

Diagram 4.4.3c: Plank with Leg Raise and Arm Lift

Side plank

Weakened QL muscles (section 4.2.6.5) can lead to recurring lower back pain. Keeping your QL strong will also help you to improve the way you perform everyday actions, such as bending from your waist. Exercises for strengthening the QL include side bends on a stability ball and side planks.

Teaching Points (Diagram 4.4.3d)

- Start by lying on your right-hand side with your legs straight. Support your upper body on your right forearm and elbow by positioning your elbow under your shoulder.

- Stack your feet, knees and thighs one on top of each other.
- Elevate your hips until your torso forms a straight line from your shoulders to your feet, ensuring that your head stays in line with your body.
- Maintain activation of your TvA, tighten your glutes, and breathe normally.
- Hold this position for as long as you can, with progression to a longer period over time. For example, start with thirty seconds and then progress to one minute, and so on. You can challenge yourself further by lifting and lowering your top leg while staying in this plank position.
- Repeat on the other side.
- If the above is too difficult, for better balance, you can start with bent knees or have both feet on the floor, one behind the other, rather than stacking them on top of each other.

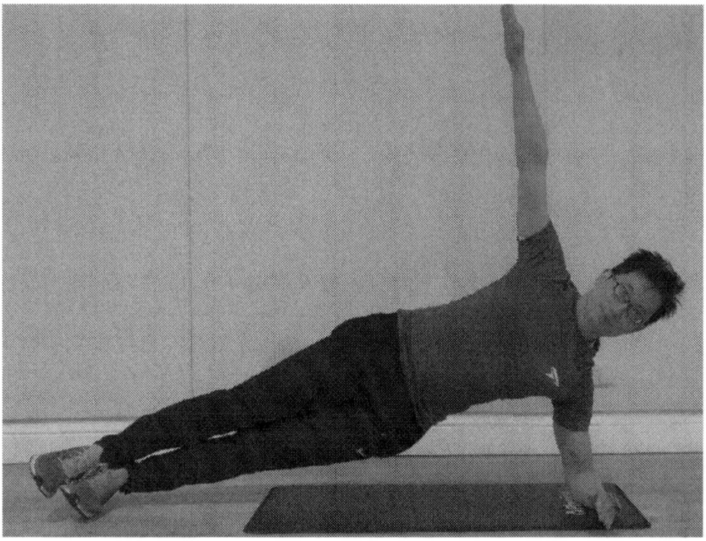

Diagram 4.4.3d: Side Plank

Plank on a Swiss (Balance) Ball

The plank on a Swiss ball is a progression from the basic plank. It can enhance your core stability (section 4.5.1) because the stabilizer muscles throughout your body are less engaged in the standard plank. This is because the stability ball is an unstable surface; when performing the plank on it, you will engage more muscles across the entire core, as well as the stabilizer muscles (section 4.5.1) from the shoulders, back and toes, which act to stabilize one joint so the desired movement can be performed in another joint. These muscles usually are not directly involved in a movement but instead work to keep you steady so that your primary muscles can do their job.

Teaching Points (Diagram 4.4.3e)

- Start by getting into the plank position, but instead of placing your forearms on the floor, place them on the Swiss ball. Place your toes on the floor as with the basic plank.
- Maintain activation of your TvA and breathe normally. Again, your body should form a straight line from your head to your toes without sagging or arching at your hips.
- Hold this position for as long as possible.
- To progress, keep your feet closer together, or even lift one foot off the floor. These moves will make balancing more difficult and challenge your core stability even further.
- To decrease the difficulty, spread your feet wide apart for a larger base of support.

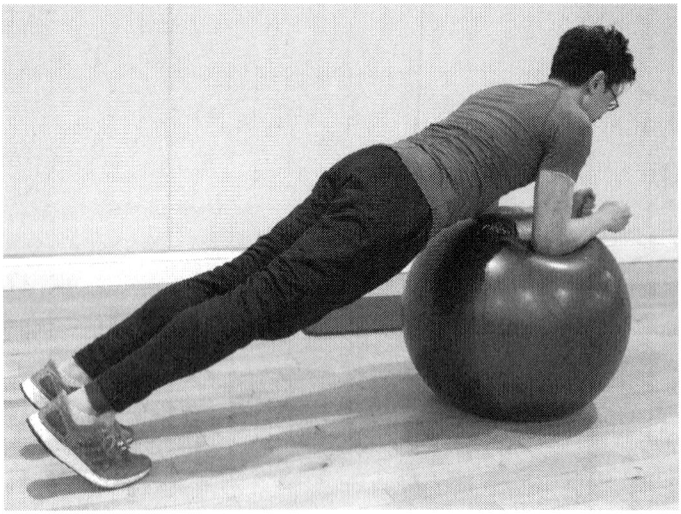

Diagram 4.4.3e: Plank on Swiss Ball

Bicycle Crunch (or elbow-to-knee twisting crunch)

Planks are isometric exercises as they do not involve any movements. It is unlikely that you will get a "washboard stomach" by only performing planks. Therefore, it is worth contemplating some other functional exercises, such as abdominal crunches, that not only involve your core musculatures, but also train your superficial muscles, such as the rectus abdominis and the obliques, strengthen them, and enhance the "six-pack" effect.

Teaching Points

- Lie on the floor on your back, with your knees raised and your hands gently supporting your head.
- Curl your right elbow towards your left knee, bringing them together over the centre of your body.
- Return to your starting position and repeat with your left elbow towards your right knee.
- Start with twenty and then progress to more repetitions.
- The exercise should be performed slowly in a controlled manner, with your TvA engaged throughout while breathing normally.

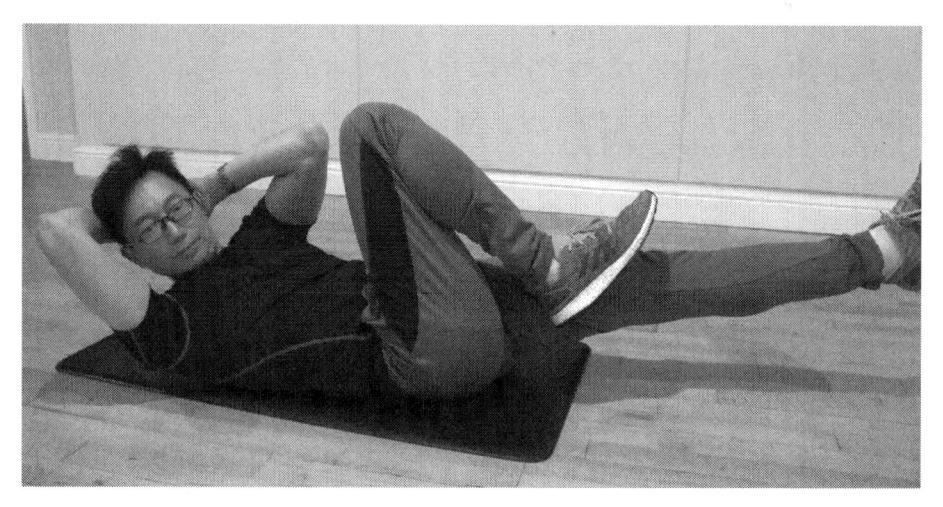

Diagram 4.4.3f: Bicycle Crunch

4.5 Integrated Dynamic Movements

As discussed in previous chapters, we tend to spend a lot of time sitting down. Besides causing muscle imbalances, our core muscles therefore become progressively weakened because we are not utilizing them to routinely stabilize our spine in our daily activities. Subconsciously, we are gradually losing the ability to activate them. As a result, other muscles overcompensate, taking on the roles of the stabilizers (see section 3.6 on synergic dominance), and this can predispose us to injury or lower back pain. To rectify these problems, the stabilizing muscles need to be retrained using core-stability exercises.

4.5.1 Core Stability

<u>What Is Core Stability?</u>

The definition of core stability is "The effective recruitment of the muscles that stabilize the lumbo-pelvic-hip complex and the spine". Core-stability exercises thus involve strengthening of the core musculatures surrounding the back and abdomen (section 3.3.2), because these muscles provide a solid base upon which all other muscles can work to initiate any functional movements. A healthy exercise routine should therefore consist of components that improve your overall cardiovascular fitness (section 5.4), muscle strength and power through resistance training (section 5.6), flexibility through stretching (section 4.3.1), and core activation through core-stability exercises.

What are stabilizer/fixator muscles (section 3.4)? The name simply describes exactly what these muscles do. They act to stabilize one joint so the desired movement can be performed in another joint. These muscles are usually not directly involved in a movement but work to keep you steady so your prime movers can perform their jobs. For example, during bicep curls, your shoulder muscles need to contract isometrically to stabilize as you curl towards the shoulders. That means just doing one exercise requires multiple muscles to fire simultaneously. Strengthening these muscles will not only help your form but will also increase your ability to balance and your coordination.

"Core stability" and "core strength" are terms that are often used interchangeably when discussing training the trunk musculature, but they are actually quite different. Training for core stability requires resisting motion at the lumbar spine through activation of the abdominal core musculature as a whole (e.g., by performing a shoulder press on a Swiss stability ball). Training for core strength allows for motions to occur through the lumbar spine in an attempt to work the abdominal musculature, often in an isolated fashion (e.g., the plank, section 4.4.3, core-strengthening exercises).

Although core stability exercises are not performed with the primary purpose of getting you fitter or shedding a few kilograms in weight, they will assist you in enhancing your core stability as well as in injury prevention, rehabilitation, and sports performance. This chapter provides you with an insight into how to explore the many different variables involved in exercise execution, progression and adaptation. Your exercise professional should be able to adapt these exercises to your own goals and requirements.

<u>Components of the Core</u>

You are reminded that the core can be considered to be a cylinder of muscles around the inner surface of the abdomen and the primary component is the four main core muscle groups (section 3.3.2.2):

Transversus Abdominis (TvA, section 4.4.2.3): This is the deepest of all the abdominal muscles; it lies under the oblique abdominals and rectus abdominis (the six-pack).

Multifidis: This deep back muscle lies on either side of the spine and again connects to each individual lumbar vertebra.

Diaphragm: The primary muscle for breathing, the domed diaphragm provides the top of the cylinder core.

Pelvic floor: The pelvic floor muscles provide a sling running from back to front, from the bottom tip of the spine (the tailbone) to the front of the pelvis.

They provide support for pelvic organs, such as the bladder and the intestines, help maintain continence, and facilitate childbirth. The pelvic floor contracts simultaneously with the TvA to form the bottom of the cylinder of muscles. These muscles can become weakened by pregnancy, childbirth, obesity, inactivity, and excessive coughing. Damage to the pelvic floor can contribute to urinary incontinence and lead to pelvic organ prolapse. Pelvic floor exercises can help to improve the tone and function of the pelvic floor muscles.

These core muscles should contract together prior to any arm or leg movement to increase intra-abdominal pressure, similar to an inflated balloon compressing upon the spine, keeping the spine in its most stable position and aiding the prevention of injury. Recent evidence has found that in people with lower back pain, these muscles fail to contract before limb movement, and so the spine is vulnerable to injury. Thus, retraining these muscles to contract at the correct time is the fundamental theory of core stability.

The rationale of core-stability training is to place the body in an "unstable" environment. The central nervous system (CNS) is able to learn how to manipulate the muscles to produce movement with the right amount of force at the right time. If the CNS is never challenged, it will never be forced to adapt and improve in its functional capacities.

Many people who go to the gym regularly fall into the trap of only paying attention to training their superficial muscles, ignoring the fact that the function of these peripheral/global muscles (section 3.3.2.3) is greatly dependent on the stability and proper functioning of the deeper core musculatures. Weakness in the core muscles requires the rest of the body to compensate, overworking other muscles and often initiating one or more trigger point cascade (section 6.2.8).

<u>Benefits of Enhancement of Core Stability</u>

- Reduced incidence of lower back injuries.
- Improved posture (e.g., activating your core musculatures can reverse your hyperlordosis and anterior pelvic tilt, section 6.3).
- Improved power, agility, speed, balance, and coordination.

The primary role of the outer unit muscles (global muscles) is to initiate movement, although some do have a stabilization role. They work in unison with the inner musculature (local muscles), which have a stiffening effect on the spine. Poor conditioning of the inner unit stabilizers can lead to spinal injury and/or back pain.

It is important to realize that core activation should be a prerequisite for all exercise programmes. Any functional movement, whether relating to a sporting action or a lifestyle activity, such as lifting a heavy item or simply walking, should be performed with the core activated.

Core Stability Exercises

Sit-Ups (section 3.3.4)

When we ask ordinary gym-goers for their opinion on the best core-stability exercise, nine out of ten will say sit-ups. They are usually under the misconception that this is a core or abdominal exercise which is effective in shedding abdominal fat. In fact, sit-ups are detrimental, because when you flex your spine excessively, you will initially be engaging your rectus abdominis, but then you will be utilizing your hip flexors to lift your lower back off the ground. The problem is that if you sit a lot, as we have discussed, your hip flexors are likely to be tight already. As the psoas major is attached to the transverse process of your T12–L5 vertebrae, this stress can aggravate the spinal discs and joints, which can be bad for your posture and can cause back pain and potentially spinal injury.

Furthermore, sit-ups are performed repetitively in an endurance-type capacity. The rectus abdominis is mainly responsible for this action, which effectively results in fast-twitch muscles taking on the role of slow-twitch muscles. This often weakens the deeper stabilizer muscles, such as the transversus abdominis. The rectus abdominis tries to perform both stabilizing and mobilizing roles, thus "switching off" the deeper core muscles, leading to back pain or injury, as optimal stabilization of the spine is not performed.

If sit-ups are not recommended as a core-stability exercise, what exercises should you do to improve stability?

The Introduction of Unstable Bases

Routine resistance training on machines (section 5.6.3) requires little stabilization control; consequently, the brain relaxes and does not engage the postural muscles, resulting in minimal functional strength gains. In other words, muscular strength and stabilization around the joints would not carry over to normal life/functional movements.

Core stability can be enhanced dramatically through the use of equipment that has an unstable base, thus requiring you to utilize your stabilization muscles to assist your balance. The more unstable your training environment, the greater the activation required for your stabilizer muscles and neutralizer muscles to maintain your centre of gravity. Stabilizer muscles are those that surround the joints and protect them from injury. The neutralizer muscles act alongside other muscles to counteract any external force that could disrupt your balance.

It should be noted that there is no single optimum exercise that can help you to achieve this powerful core; instead, a balance of exercises appropriate to your own goals and specific needs is required. This is why you are advised to seek help from an exercise professional who will not only introduce you to these exercises but also monitor your progress and alter the variables to make the exercises more challenging. Generally speaking, your training programme should incorporate core stabilization training with or without functional movements at least three times a week.

Examples of "unstable" equipment (see diagram 4.5.1a below) include the gym stability (Swiss) ball, the Reebok Core Board, and the BOSU ball. Once you have been taught the correct exercise techniques by your exercise professional, you can perform these exercises at home or at work.

When choosing your Swiss/stability ball, you should ensure that it is large enough so that when seated on it with your feet together and your thighs parallel to the floor, your knees are at an approximately ninety-degree angle. The ball should be relatively firm, because the firmer the ball, the more difficult the exercises will be.

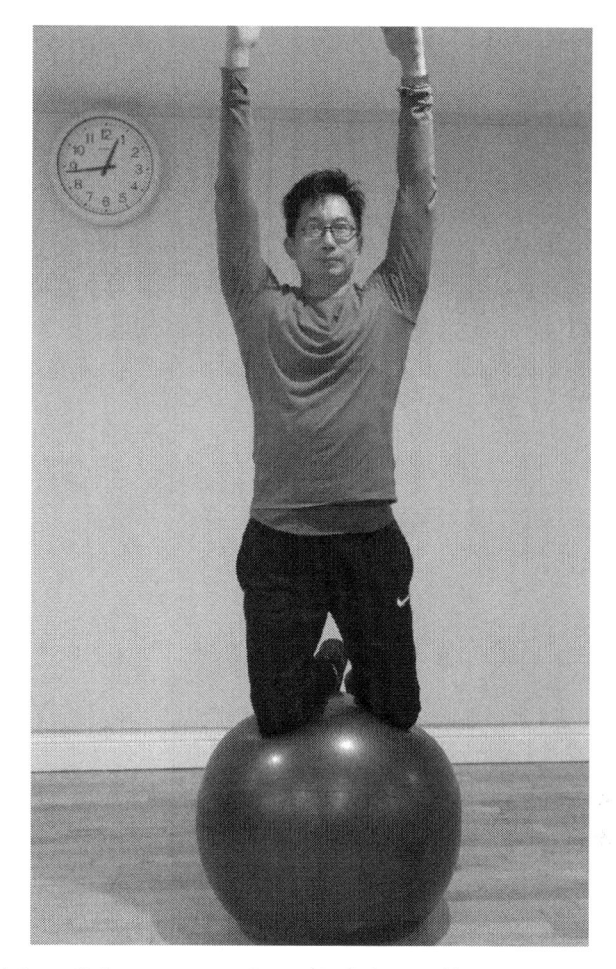

Diagram 4.5.1a: Balancing on a Swiss/Stability Ball

As with any exercises, it is important to warm up (section 5.4.1) through joint mobilization and dynamic stretching (section 5.6.1) prior to your main exercise session.

Stabilization Exercises with Conventional Training

It is advisable to use multi-joint exercises in all planes of motion (frontal, saggital, and transverse) from both a bilateral and unilateral stance to help increase muscle synergy and re-educate the neuromuscular system to maintain proper postural alignment during functional activities. These exercises should involve low load and controlled movement in an ideal posture to ensure that joints start and remain in proper alignment, muscles function in their proper length-tension relationships, and synergistic muscle recruitment is optimal.

For instance, you can improve your core stability by performing some of your routine exercises, such as abdominal crunches, back extensions, bicep curls, and shoulder or chest presses (see diagram 4.5.1b below) on a Swiss ball. You may have to drop your weight, as besides engaging the prime movers (section 3.4), you need to engage your core to stabilize yourself on the ball.

Other examples include single-leg stance exercises on a wobble plate. Keep your eyes open at first and then progress to performing the exercises with eyes closed in order to challenge your proprioception even further.

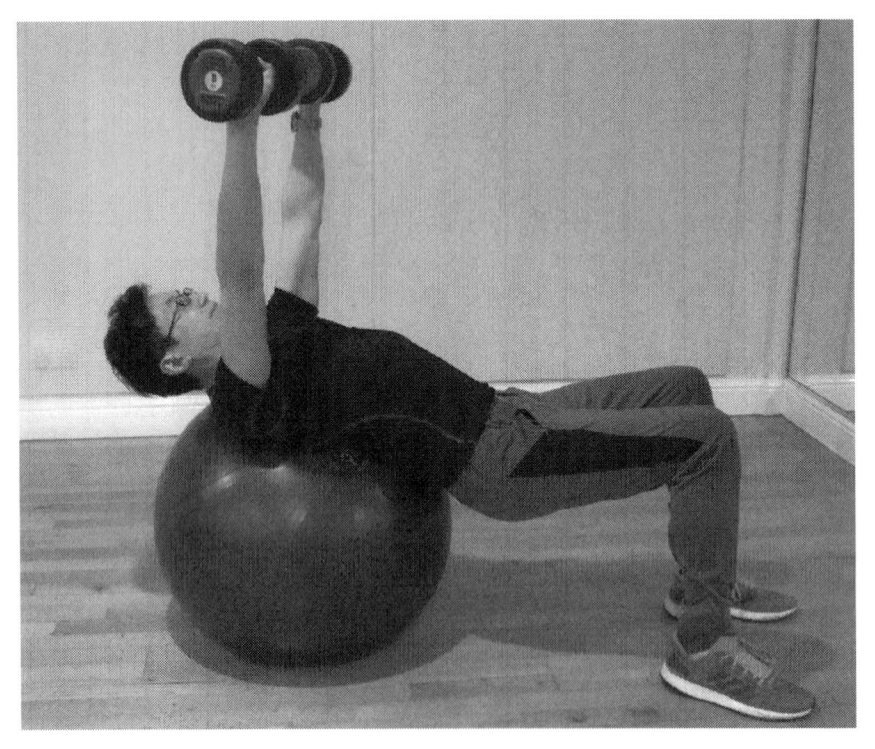

Diagram 4.5.1b: Chest Press on Swiss Ball

Summary

As with any new exercise routine, always check with your doctor, exercise professional, or physiotherapist to confirm there are no contraindications that might prevent you from embarking on a new training programme. Conditions such as acute injury, muscle strain or tear of the muscle being worked on, acute rheumatoid arthritis of the affected joints, etc. may cause pain in certain positions. Additionally, it is important to identify any imbalances you may have and introduce corrective exercises to recondition any muscles that may restrict your progression.

Please be aware that there are no quick-fix solutions, especially with these core exercises; they need to be learnt through regular practice because the more you do, the more efficient your brain becomes in instructing these muscles to work, enhancing your neuromuscular efficiency. Unlike the results from resistance training, it may take many months before you will notice any benefits from these core exercises, and you need to be patient.

It is beyond the scope of this book to go through the details and teaching points of every single unstable surface exercise. There are numerous online tutorials that demonstrate the correct techniques for these activities. The purpose of this chapter is simply to highlight the rationale and importance of using unstable exercises to enhance your core stability as part of the holistic management of your lower back pain. In order to achieve maximal benefits, it is imperative that you engage an exercise professional who can devise a complete and bespoke programme for you (such as the repetition range and number of sets per exercise) and guide you through these exercises.

Generally speaking, however, core exercises target type 1 postural fibres (section 2.3); these are endurance exercises. You should do three to six sets of twelve to twenty repetitions when performing these exercises.

For your information, a repetition range from one to six is for power, a range from six to twelve is for hypertrophy, and a range from twelve upwards is for endurance (section 5.6.2). You can perform four to five sets on average.

CHAPTER 5

Obesity and Back Pain

5.1 Introduction to Obesity and Back Pain

In this chapter, we will look at the effect of obesity on back problems and explore the various ways that you can shed weight effectively. This is not a textbook on nutrition, and the objective of this chapter is to provide a simplistic and generalized overview of the macronutrients that are relevant to exercise and weight loss.

The spine is designed to carry the body's weight and distribute the loads encountered during rest and activity. When excess weight is carried, the spine is forced to assimilate the burden, predisposing the body to structural compromise and damage. The area of the spine that is most vulnerable to the effects of obesity is the lower back (lumbar spine).

As already discussed, sitting for prolonged periods can lead to muscle imbalances, predisposing us to back problems (section 3.6). Furthermore, working for long hours and a lack of physical activity cause weight gain, especially abdominal obesity, which shifts the centre of gravity forward. This in turn leads to an increased chance of hyperlordosis and anterior pelvic tilt (section 6.2.1). Such postural deviations can lead to faulty loading patterns, which increase the strain on the spine and surrounding joint structures. Those with hyperlordosis often have a reduced range of lumbar flexion and restricted mobility, thereby increasing the risk of disc injuries which can cause nerves to be pinched, resulting in pain, such as sciatica (section 4.3.2.5).

Is Back Pain Related to Age?

You may try to dismiss the cause of some of these spinal disorders as part of the normal process of ageing. It is true that with age, body tissues can cause changes to spinal anatomy; however, if you are overweight or obese, the chances are that you may have developed one of the following conditions:

- **Postural problems:** These include hyperlordosis and anterior pelvic tilt.
- **Lower back pain:** Obesity may aggravate an existing lower back problem and contribute to a recurrence of the condition.
- **Osteoporosis:** A sedentary lifestyle coupled with an unbalanced diet can affect the density and hence the strength of your bones. When the structural architecture of a spinal vertebral body is compromised, it is at risk of fracture, which can be both painful and disabling.
- **Osteoarthritis (OA) and rheumatoid arthritis (RA):** Excessive body weight places unnatural pressure and stress on the facet joints of the spine during movement and while at rest.

Are You Overweight or Obese?

If you are overweight or obese, there are many ways of losing weight and maintaining a healthier body composition. To get started, talk with your doctor or a fitness professional to establish your ultimate goals (which must be realistic and achievable, section 5.6) and determine how you can safely begin a sustainable weight-loss programme. This is important because if you suffer from back pain, your exercise programme is likely to be different from that of someone without such problems. Remember: no two people are the same, and obtaining professional help is the best initial step.

James Tang

Does Cardiovascular Exercise Help You Lose Weight?

Whilst physical activity is useful in reducing the risk of certain diseases, it does not necessarily promote weight loss. A person who exercises often cancels out the calories they have burned by eating more, generally as a form of self-reward. In order to understand the physiology of weight loss, we need to understand the relationships between diet, metabolism (section 5.2), and the circumstances under which the body begins to burn fat as fuel (section 5.3).

5.2 Metabolism and Macronutrients

Metabolism is the sum of all the biochemical processes that occur in the body, including:

- Anabolism, the formation of larger molecules, and
- Catabolism, the breakdown of larger molecules into smaller ones.

The body's rate of energy expenditure is the metabolic rate, and the total caloric expenditure is the product of a number of interacting factors:

- The basal metabolic rate (BMR) is the total sum of all the reactions that occur in the body when at complete rest with no digestion occurring. This is usually expressed as the number of calories needed to sustain basic functioning.
- The thermic effect of food is the amount of energy expended by the body through the ingestion, digestion, absorption, utilization, and storage of food. This accounts for 6–10 per cent of daily energy expenditure for men and 6–7 per cent for women.
- The thermic effect of activity is the amount of energy required for planned and unplanned levels of physical activities. This is the most variable component of energy expenditure, and it accounts for approximately 20–40 per cent of total energy expenditure.

| Metabolic Rate = BMR + Thermic Effect of Food + Thermic Effect of Activity |

One gram of these different food components produces the following energy values:

- Carbohydrate—4 kcal
- Fat—9 kcal
- Protein—4 kcal
- Alcohol—7 kcal

Weight control is simply a matter of creating an energy imbalance which forces your body to burn fat stores for energy. The energy balance equation requires consideration of both energy intake (food and drink) and energy expenditure (basal metabolic rate, thermic effect of food, and physical activity). In simple terms, if you take in more calories than your total caloric expenditure, you put on weight. If you expend more than you take in, you lose weight. Whether these calories come from readily accessible calories or fat stores, you are going to burn fat as long as you maintain a calorie deficit, which can be achieved when you reduce your caloric intake, increase your level of physical activity, or do a combination of both. No matter which method you use, if you eat fewer calories than you need, your body will access fat stores for energy.

For the purpose of weight loss, only macronutrients (carbohydrates, proteins, and fats), which are used to fuel body activities, will be considered in this book. It must be emphasized that it is important that you maintain a balanced diet which also includes the recommended levels of micronutrients (vitamins, minerals).

The Eatwell Plate (Diagram 5.2) highlights the various types of food that make up our diet and shows the proportions we should eat them in to have a healthy, balanced diet.

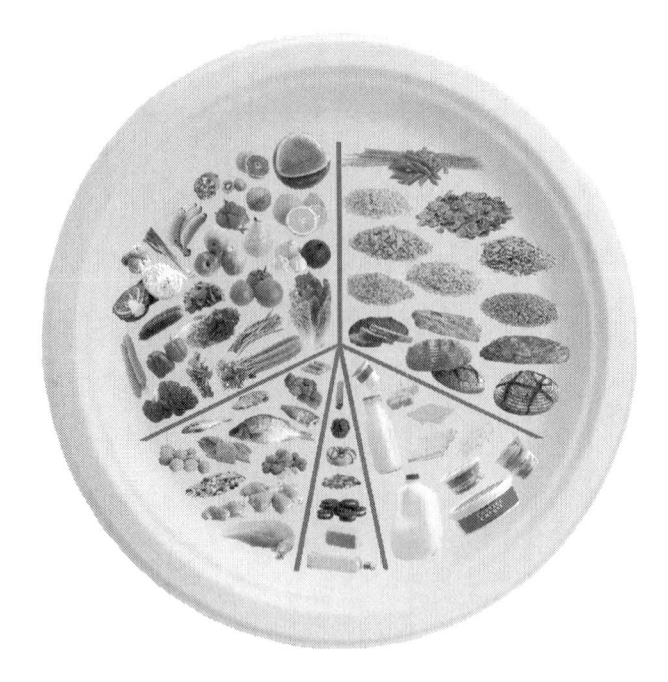

Diagram 5.2: The Eatwell Plate

It's a good idea to try to get this balance right every day, but does not need to be done at every meal. You may find it easier to get the balance right over a longer period—a week, for example. Whenever possible, try to choose options that are low in salt.

Energy Intake from Macronutrients

5.2.1 Carbohydrates

Carbohydrates are stored as glycogen in the muscles and liver. There is approximately three times more glycogen stored in the muscles than in the liver. Increasing your muscle mass will also increase your storage capacity for glycogen. On average, the total store of glycogen is about five hundred grams, which is equivalent to sixteen hundred to two thousand kilocalories—enough to last a day if you were to eat nothing. This is why a low-carbohydrate diet tends to make people lose quite a lot of weight in the first few days; this weight loss is almost entirely due to the loss of glycogen and water.

On average, you have enough intramuscular glycogen to fuel 90–180 minutes of endurance activity; the higher the intensity, the faster your muscle glycogen stores will be depleted. The greater your pre-exercise muscle glycogen store, the longer you will be able to maintain your exercise intensity and delay the onset of fatigue.

The glycaemic index (GI) is the speed at which you digest food and convert it into glucose. Glucose has a glycaemic index of one hundred. If you need to get carbohydrates into your bloodstream and muscle cells rapidly (e.g., immediately after exercise to replenish your glycogen), you should choose high-GI food.

It is, however, not advisable to eat high-GI food before exercise. When glucose levels are high, large amounts of insulin are produced, which shunts the excess glucose into fat cells, leading to transient hypoglycaemia. The safest strategy, therefore, is to consume low-GI food before exercise and then top up with high-GI carbohydrates during or shortly after exercise.

To optimize glycogen storage and minimize fat storage, aim to achieve a small or moderate glycaemic load. Eat little and often, and avoid overloading on carbohydrates. There is, however, no need to cut out food with a high glycaemic index. The key is to eat high-GI food with protein and/or a little healthy fat, which will slow down the release of glucose.

Apples (despite containing simple carbohydrates) generate a small and prolonged rise in blood sugar. A great deal of starch-rich food (complex carbohydrates), such as potatoes and bread, is digested and absorbed very quickly and causes a rapid rise in blood sugar.

It is not a good idea at all to try and lose weight by combining a low-calorie diet with a lengthy cardio workout. This is because (1) your body adapts so you have to do more to get the same result, and (2) as low-calorie diets tend to be low in carbohydrates, once you have used up your intramuscular glycogen, the body starts to metabolize protein for energy. So not only are you not losing fat, but you are also losing muscle mass. This is detrimental because whilst we think that we expend most of our calories when we are exercising, most of our energy is used up simply existing, even if you do nothing for twenty-four hours, you will still be burning nearly seventeen hundred calories in a day (basal metabolic rate), and the more muscle mass you have, the more calories you burn whilst you rest. This is why building muscle is an effective way of burning fat (section 5.6).

5.2.2 Fats

Some fat is necessary since it cushions our internal organs, helps us to assimilate vitamins, and stores energy for use later on. Unlike muscles, fat does not burn calories; it stores them. Although one kilogram of fat weighs exactly the same as one kilogram of muscle, fat takes up more room than muscle, which increases our overall size.

Fat is stored as adipose tissue in almost every region of the body. A small amount of fat, about three hundred to four hundred grams, is stored in muscles as intramuscular fat. The majority is stored around the organs and beneath the skin. People who have abdominal obesity with the classic pot-belly shape are known to have a higher risk of heart disease than those who store fat mostly around their hips and thighs (pear shape).

You cannot do anything about the way your body distributes fat, but you can change the amount of fat that is stored. Female hormones tend to favour fat storage around the hips and thighs, whilst male hormones encourage fat storage around the middle.

It is a general misconception by most people that abdominal exercises, such as abdominal crunches or sit-ups are effective in removing your abdominal fat. Let us be clear: no exercise on its own can remove your belly fat. The key to losing belly fat is self-motivation to exercise regularly, eating a balanced and healthy diet, reducing stress, and consuming more calories than you take in.

The more overall body weight you lose, the more quickly you will start losing your belly fat. That said, you should not aim for a massive weight reduction within a short period of time as this is unrealistic and unsustainable. It is much better to lose weight gradually.

5.2.3 Protein

Protein is primarily used as a building material rather than as an energy store. However, it can be broken down to release energy if necessary—for example, during very prolonged (usually in excess of an hour) or very intense bouts of exercise, when glycogen stores become depleted. Some people think that if they deplete their glycogen stores by following a low-carbohydrate diet, they will force their body to break down more fat and lose weight. This is not always the case, as we have mentioned above, as you risk losing muscle as well as fat.

Exercise triggers the activation of an enzyme that oxidizes key amino acids in the muscle, which are then used as a fuel source. The greater the exercise intensity and the longer its duration, the more protein is broken down for fuel. Therefore, if you are following a weight-loss programme, do not reduce your carbohydrates too drastically; otherwise, protein will be used as an energy source, making it unavailable for tissue growth. A higher protein intake can offset some of the associated muscle-wasting effects.

5.2.3.1 Protein Supplements

The bioavailability of a particular protein is often measured by its biological value (BV). For example, an egg has a BV of 100. Whey proteins are extracted from curdled milk. They have a BV of up to 159, which is considerably higher than that of an egg.

Many protein shakes contain whey protein, which is found in milk, and has the highest biological value to the body of any protein. The problem is that whey powder in protein supplements is often dried at high temperatures during the manufacturing process, and at above sixty degrees Celsius, these fragile proteins become denatured, subsequently destroying their ability to function. Furthermore, manufacturers often use sweeteners, colouring, and flavour to improve the palatability of these supplements. These products are often very low in fat, but fat needs to be present for protein to be metabolized and used. Generally speaking, protein supplements are harmless but unnecessary.

For building muscle mass, an overall daily protein intake of 1.4-2.0 grams of protein per kilogram body weight per day is adequate for most individuals. It is much better to obtain protein from whole food sources, such as eggs, fish, chicken, etc.

<u>Summary</u>

You fuel your workout with carbohydrates, fats and proteins, but carbohydrates are the body's preferred energy source, as they are the easiest to burn. In the absence of carbohydrates, the body burns fat, and then protein. The amount of carbohydrates consumed during exercise depends on the type, duration, and intensity of the exercise.

Weight control is a matter of creating an energy imbalance, i.e., if you take in more calories than your total caloric expenditure, you put on weight. If you expend more than you take in, you lose weight. In the next part (section 5.3), we will take a look at the physiology of how the body burns fat as fuel and how we can optimize fat burning in a holistic weight-loss programme.

5.3 The Energy Systems

To understand the effects of exercises on the body's system, we need to analyse how the body creates energy for these activities, and how the different forms of exercise and their level of intensity place different demands on energy production. In order to understand the most effective way of burning fat, we need to understand how our body acquires energy in the first place.

All functions of the body require energy, and this energy comes from the breakdown of adenosine triphosphate (ATP). There is a limited store of ATP within the muscle, and it lasts only for approximately one or two seconds. Re-synthesis of ATP comes from either the breakdown of phosphocreatine or macronutrients in the diet, such as carbohydrates, fats, and proteins.

Creatine is produced in the liver from amino acids and it is transported in the blood to muscle cells, where it is combined with phosphate to make phosphocreatine. Creatine can be obtained in the diet from fish. Vegetarians have no dietary source of creatine.

Adenosine triphosphate (ATP) is made up of one adenosine and three phosphate molecules. When one of these phosphates is removed, the energy is released. This is a crucial reaction to sustain life. When one of the three phosphates is removed, the resulting compound is called adenosine diphosphate (ADP). ADP can be converted back into ATP so that it can be used again. ATP is constantly being used by the body so it needs to be re-synthesized regularly. The three energy systems use different fuels to convert ADP back into ATP.

5.3.1 Creatine Phosphate, or Phosphocreatine, System (CP System)

The CP system is anaerobic and does not require oxygen, fats, or carbohydrates. ATP can be regenerated almost immediately using creatine phosphate, but again, this lasts only for a very short period of time because of the limited creatine phosphate store. The CP system is exhausted after a maximum of ten seconds. This energy system is used during activities requiring maximal exertion and when muscles need to generate a lot of force very quickly (e.g., a one-hundred-metre sprint).

CP and ATP stores are 50 per cent restored after thirty seconds and fully restored after about five minutes of rest.

5.3.2 Lactate System

The lactate system uses intramuscular glycogen (carbohydrates) to make ATP. Glycogen is broken down into glucose without oxygen. One glucose molecule produces two ATP molecules along with lactic acid as a waste product.

This system is used when near maximal exercise lasts longer than CP sources can sustain activity (beyond ten seconds) or when the intensity during aerobic activity starts to demand more energy than the aerobic system can provide.

When the production of lactic acid exceeds the body's ability to disperse it, there will be a build-up of lactic acid—onset of blood lactate accumulation (OBLA). Targeted interval training improves this lactate tolerance (section 5.5).

Anaerobic training uses up the intramuscular glycogen store after one to three minutes. Recovery should be active (e.g., walking between running intervals) to aid the return of blood to the liver. This is known as 'active rest'.

5.3.3 Aerobic System

The aerobic system involves the production of ATP from the complete breakdown of carbohydrates, fats and proteins in the presence of oxygen. This system is active when there is sufficient oxygen to meet the demand of energy production (e.g., when the body is at rest and the intensity of the activity is low to moderate).

Carbohydrates are the preferred energy source, because they will release energy a lot faster, although they release less energy per molecule than fat.

The aerobic system produces ATP, carbon dioxide, water, and heat from the breakdown of fats and carbohydrates.

Surprisingly, the best way to burn fat is actually with light exercise (60–70 per cent of your maximum heart rate, section 5.4.2). This will typically burn high percentages of fat. Fat burns slowly as fuel and requires oxygen to burn properly. However, lighter exercises also burn fewer overall calories. People who perform more intense exercises will lose more calories, but without sufficient oxygen getting to their cells, they will not lose fat quite as quickly and will instead lose carbohydrates.

Whilst it is convenient to describe the systems as separate concepts, during actual exercises, all three systems interweave to produce the desired performance outcome. It is the intensity of the exercise that dictates which one will be used to supply the majority of the energy.

5.3.4 How Does Diet Contribute to Weight Loss?

The total amount of calories should be divided across each of the macronutrients to achieve the following recommended ratios:

- Minimum of 50 per cent of total calories from carbohydrates
- Maximum of 35 per cent of total calories from fats
- Minimum of 55 grams of protein per day (approximately 10 per cent of total calories)

You must have seen people who have dropped a lot of weight, but who look tired and unwell. With drastic calorie drops, increases in expenditure create a massive stress on the body. If you are spending hours doing cardio exercises on low calories, and your performance in your session is suffering dramatically, then this should be your wake-up call. Other undesirable drastic diet effects include loss of sex drive, irritability, poor quality of sleep and constantly feeling hungry etc.

Therefore, the key to successful fat loss is to cut your fat to approximately 25 per cent of your total calories and to reduce carbohydrates only modestly. Ideally, carbohydrates should continue to contribute about 50 per cent of your total calories. Reducing your usual calorie intake by a modest amount of about 15 per cent will avoid the metabolic slowdown that is associated with more severe calorie reduction. The body will recognize and react to a small deficit by oxidizing more fat. If you cut calories more drastically, you will not shed fat faster. Instead, this will cause your body to lower its metabolic rate in an attempt to conserve energy. It will also increase the breakdown of protein and depletion of glycogen, resulting in loss of muscle tissue, low energy levels, and extreme hunger.

It is therefore recommended that you consume food more frequently and, most importantly, that you do not skip breakfast. Every time we eat, the metabolic rate increases by approximately 10 per cent for a short while afterwards, owing to the thermic effect of food. Furthermore, frequent eating keeps blood sugar and insulin levels more stable.

5.3.5 How Does Stress Affect Your Weight?

Cortisol, the primary corticosteroid released from the adrenal cortex, helps to provide reserves in the body for managing stress. It is a catabolic hormone which promotes the breakdown of carbohydrates, proteins, and fats to provide energy for the body during stressful periods. It offers support during short-term bouts of stress. Long-term chronic stress and the resulting excess cortisol can lead to deterioration in health due to an unbalancing of the endocrine system. Apart from causing muscles to break down, cortisol also causes the body to hold on to fat and boost appetite. It encourages fat to be stored around the middle, and it is known that fat in this area is associated with an increased risk of heart disease and diabetes.

5.3.6 Diet and Exercise

Please note that only general advice is given here, and it is not specific to any individual person. You should consult your exercise professional or nutritionist for a bespoke exercise and nutrition plan devised in accordance with your specific goals.

<u>When Is the Best Time to Eat before Exercise?</u>

Eat approximately two hours before training, as this leaves ample time for your stomach to settle so that you feel comfortable and not too hungry. If fat loss is your main goal, exercising on an empty stomach—such as first thing in the morning—may encourage your body to burn slightly more fat for fuel, but you may fatigue sooner as a result of deprivation of your intramuscular glycogen, or you may drop your exercise intensity and therefore end up burning fewer calories. You should therefore consume 2.5 grams of carbohydrates per kilogram of body weight approximately two hours before exercise.

<u>During Exercise</u>

Generally speaking, for activities lasting less than an hour, drinking water will be adequate. For activities that are longer than an hour at moderate to high intensity, consuming carbohydrates (e.g., a glucose drink) during your workout can help delay fatigue. Consuming a drink containing protein as well as carbohydrates during exercise may minimize protein and muscle breakdown following exercise.

After Exercise

The best time to replenish your glycogen store is during the first two hours after exercise, using carbohydrates with a moderate or high GI. Eating carbohydrates stimulates insulin release, which in turn increases the amount of glucose taken up by your muscle cells from the bloodstream. Furthermore, the muscle cell membranes are more permeable to glucose after exercise so they can take up more glucose than normal. Combining carbohydrates with protein is more effective in promoting glycogen recovery than carbohydrates alone. One part of protein to three parts of carbohydrate promotes faster glycogen refuelling, muscle repair, and growth compared to an intake of carbohydrates alone.

Summary

The key to successful fat loss is to cut your total calories by reducing fat consumption but by reducing carbohydrates by only a modest amount; eat more frequently, and do not skip breakfast.

5.4 Exercises for Weight Loss: Cardiovascular Exercises

Introduction

Running on a treadmill for about sixty minutes at a steady pace results in initial weight loss, but after a few weeks, the body adapts and becomes more efficient, so the same exercise requires less effort and the rate of weight loss decreases. It is therefore best to vary your workouts in terms of length and intensity and allow a recovery day between days of training.

However, you should not exclusively rely on aerobic exercise. You could still lose substantial amounts of muscle tissue with aerobic exercise because these exercises do not act as sufficient stimuli to ensure muscle retention.

So Which Exercise Is Best for Losing Weight?

When it comes to weight loss, anything that builds muscle is advisable, so resistance training should be included as part of your workout. Not only will this help to slow the process of sarcopenia, the loss of skeletal muscle mass due to ageing, but combining resistance training with aerobic exercises can also help to reduce abdominal fat whilst increasing or preserving muscle mass. This is because extra muscle helps to burn more energy at rest. This is called the resting metabolic rate of muscle (RMR). Extra muscle will also burn more fat in the active phase, so having more muscle will definitely help to burn more energy and fat.

A weight-training programme, however, may not burn as many calories as a cardiovascular workout, so it makes sense to increase your total caloric expenditure through some form of cardiovascular activities, such as high-intensity interval training (section 5.5). Furthermore, selecting the correct type of cardiovascular exercises can enhance your aerobic and anaerobic base, enabling you to perform your resistance training more effectively.

Cardiovascular Session

5.4.1 Warm-Up

A gradual warm-up is beneficial and can help prepare the body for more intense exercise. In fact, the more intense your exercise, event, or training routine is, the more important a proper warm-up becomes.

The cardiovascular session should follow on from the warm-up, which can involve the same type of cardiovascular equipment. At the end of the warm-up, the heart rate should be at the level required for the main cardiovascular session (see diagram 5.4.1).

The length of time spent warming up depends on the individual. If you attend a gym regularly, the warm-up does not need to be too long. For an older person not used to exercise (a deconditioned individual), the warm-up needs to be longer—up to twenty minutes. However, in general, a five-minute warm-up is adequate.

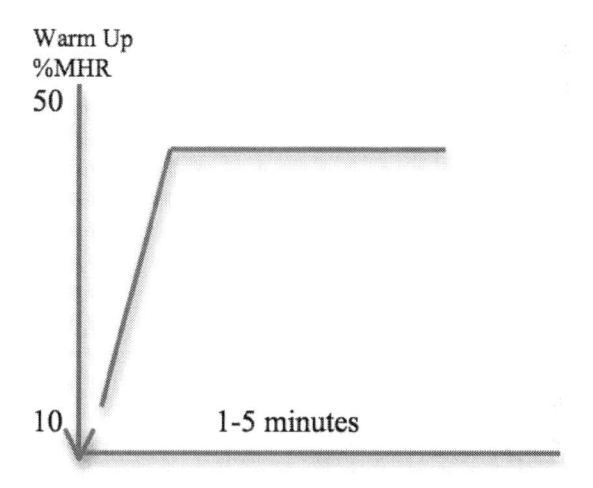

Diagram 5.4.1: Warm-Up

The ideal equipment for warming up includes cross trainers and rowing machines, which enable you to warm up your entire body (upper and lower limbs). These are more preferable than treadmills, which primarily warm up the muscles of your legs. To do a warm-up, increase the heart rate to 50 per cent of MHR (maximum heart rate, see section 5.4.2 below) in the first minute and maintain it at that rate for a further four minutes.

Benefits of Warm-Ups

- **Increased muscle temperature:** A warmed muscle contracts forcefully and relaxes quickly. In this way, both speed and strength can be enhanced.
- **Increased body temperature:** This improves muscle elasticity and reduces the risk of injury.
- **Increased blood temperature:** As blood temperature rises, the binding of oxygen to haemoglobin weakens, making oxygen is more readily available to the working muscles, which can improve endurance.
- **Improved range of motion:** The range of motion around a joint is increased through muscles being more elastic and synovial fluids being released into the joints.
- **Vasodilation:** This reduces both peripheral resistance to blood flow and stress on the heart.
- **Improved efficient cooling:** By activating the heat-dissipation mechanisms in the body (sweating), you can cool efficiently and help prevent overheating.
- **Increased secretion of hormones:** When performing a warm-up routine, additional hormones are released to provide your body with energy via additional carbohydrates and fatty acids.
- **Mental preparation: During** a warm-up routine, the mind will enter a state of focus and preparation which is required for the exercises that you are about to perform.

5.4.2 Cardio Training Zones

Are you exercising at the right intensity? Using heart rate zones allows you to tailor your cardio workout to the best intensity to fulfil your goals.

To be effective, cardiovascular exercise relies on frequency, intensity and duration. You know how often you exercise and for how long, but you also need to know your heart rate to judge your intensity. Using heart-rate zones allows you to tailor your cardio workout to the best intensity in order to fulfil your goals.

These zones relate to the heart-rate range in which certain benefits might be expected. They are not exact but are useful as a guide to cardiovascular training, as the benefits relating to each zone are reasonably accurate.

If you know your maximum heart rate (MHR), you can use heart-zone training to gear your workout to the correct intensity. Your maximum heart rate is as fast as your heart can beat. This varies for each person, but age is generally used as a guide for what your maximum heart rate is likely to be, using the formula MHR = 220 - age. However, this formula is too general and cannot represent each individual, because this MHR is the same for everyone of the same age, irrespective of their levels of fitness.

The Karvonen method of calculating your exercise heart rate is much better—especially for those who are looking for weight loss and fitness improvement. As a person becomes fitter, his or her heart becomes more efficient at pumping blood to the rest of the body. The resting heart rate therefore slows down. The Karvonen formula takes this into consideration by introducing a number called the heart rate reserve (the difference between the maximum heart rate and the resting heart rate) into the equation.

To find out what your more accurate target heart rate should be while exercising, you will need to determine your resting heart rate. The best time to check your resting rate is just before you get out of bed in the morning. Take the average of two or three mornings' readings for greater accuracy.

> 220 - age = MHR
> MHR - RHR (resting heart rate) = HRR (heart rate reserve)
> HRR × 60% (assuming a 60% cardio training zone) + RHR = MHR (specific to that individual)

For example, below is how to work out the HR training zone for a forty-year-old with a resting heart rate of seventy beats per minute.

> 220 - 40 = 180
> 180 - 70 (RHR) = 110 (HRR)
> (110 × 70%) + 70 (RHR) = 147. So this is the HR to which the individual should be trained in order to achieve a 70% cardio training zone.

Moderate Aerobic Zone: 50–60 Per Cent MHR

This is an easy and comfortable zone to exercise in and is mainly suitable for deconditioned individuals. Although you may be breathing a little heavier than usual while in this zone, you will be able to have a full conversation. Regular exercise in this zone will trigger slight improvements in cardiovascular functions. The goal is to sustain a minimum of twenty minutes before progressing to higher intensity levels.

Weight-Management Zone: 60–70 Per Cent MHR

Training within this range develops both endurance and aerobic capacity; more fat is burned at a higher rate than in the previous zone, and it is therefore effective for weight loss. More calories are burned per minute because the exercise is a little more intense. You are going faster and therefore covering more distance. The calories burned depend on the distance you cover and your weight. At this intensity, you will be breathing heavier but will still be able to speak in short sentences.

The American College of Sports Medicine (ACSM) guidelines suggest training for twenty to sixty minutes at a frequency of three to five days per week. Clearly, a greater amount of energy will be expended at 70 per cent of MHR compared to that expended at 60 per cent for the same amount of time; this will affect the overall amount of fat used as fuel for the exercise.

Aerobic Zone: 70–80 Per Cent MHR

Training in this zone will develop your cardiovascular system. The body's ability to transport oxygen to, and carbon dioxide away from, the working muscles can be developed and improved. So this is the "fitness" zone at moderate-to-vigorous intensity. You will be breathing very hard and able to speak only in short phrases. This is the zone to aim for when training for endurance. It spurs your body to improve your circulatory system by building new blood vessels and increases your heart and lung capacity.

This level is more appropriate for individuals who are used to exercising on a regular basis. As you become fitter and stronger through training in this zone, it will be possible to get the benefits of some fat burning and improved aerobic capacity.

Anaerobic Zone: 80–90 Per Cent MHR

Training in this zone will develop your lactic acid system, because your anaerobic threshold is normally reached here. You will be unable to speak except for a single gasped word at a time. With these heart rates, the amount of fat being utilized as the main source of energy is greatly reduced and glycogen stored in the muscle is predominantly used. One of the by-products of burning this glycogen is lactic acid. There is a point at which the body can no longer remove the lactic acid from the working muscles quickly enough. This is your anaerobic threshold. Through correct training, it is possible to improve your lactate tolerance by being able to increase your ability to deal with the lactic acid for a longer period of time or by pushing the anaerobic threshold higher. The greater the intensity, the greater the anaerobic contribution (section 5.3.2).

Please be aware that regardless of the exercise, all three energy systems (section 5.3) contribute to the production of energy to some extent throughout the duration of the exercise. The amount of contribution, however, depends upon the intensity of the exercise. Therefore, one must remember that even during high-intensity events, a good contribution from the aerobic system is required in addition to a contribution from the anaerobic system.

5.5 Exercises for Weight Loss: High-Intensity Interval Training (HIIT)

Introduction

We are all too aware of the importance of regular exercise for healthy living, and are also well informed about the adverse effect of obesity due to a sedentary lifestyle. Furthermore, we also know that prolonged sitting is related to a whole host of musculoskeletal disorders, such as lower back pain and neck pain. Of course, we would all wish to enhance our cardiovascular fitness and well-being through regular exercise; the problem is, for most people, fitness training comprises a workout involving a long, continuous, and boring routine at a constant intensity. In this day and age when everyone is so busy, we do not always have time to spend hour after hour in the gym, so what is the most effective way of burning fat and improving overall fitness? Well, according to the American College of Sports Medicine (ACSM), more calories are burned in short, high-intensity exercise routines. So, HIIT provides similar fitness benefits to routine endurance workouts but in a shorter period of time. Not only does this type of training improve our overall cardiovascular fitness and save time, it also helps us to increase our metabolism and hence burn calories for hours after we have completed our workout.

What Is Interval Training?

Athletes have used interval training to build fitness for many years. This type of training combines short, high-intensity bursts of speed with slow recovery phases (active rest), repeated during one exercise session. An early form of interval training, "fartlek" (a Swedish term meaning "speed play"), was casual and unstructured. A runner would simply increase and decrease his pace at will. Today athletes use more structured interval training workouts to build speed and endurance.

The Energy Systems

You already learnt in section 5.2 that all functions of the body require energy, which comes from the breakdown of adenosine triphosphate

(ATP). Your metabolism is how your body converts the nutrients you consume in your diet into ATP (section 5.3).

Why Use High-Intensity Interval Training?

It was believed that a long, steady-paced cardio workout was superior for fat loss because relatively more fat is burned via aerobic glycolysis (section 5.3.3) at lower exercise intensities than at higher intensities. The so-called "weight-management or fat-burning zone" (section 5.4.2), which is around 60–70 per cent of the maximum heart rate, is not necessarily optimal for burning fat. It is true that fat calories are burned during prolonged low-intensity exercise, but fewer overall calories are burned during this type of exercise. It is also a fact that you burn more fat relative to glycogen, but the main concern is the aggregate amount of fat burned. At higher intensities, you burn more fat in total, even though the fat-glycogen ratio is lower. Essentially, the total amount of calories you burn is more important than which calories are burned. The number of calories burned depends on the distance you cover, so the more intense your training, the greater the duration, and the greater the frequency, the more calories will be expended, as you will be covering a greater distance.

- One gram of carbohydrate produces four kilocalories. Carbohydrates are converted into energy the quickest so the human body relies heavily on the easy access of stored carbohydrates as its main energy source.
- One gram of fat produces nine kilocalories. Fat is not as readily available as carbohydrates; it must go through additional processes before being converted into energy.
- One gram of protein produces four kilocalories. Protein contributes very little energy.

In that case, why don't we just push hard the whole time instead of mixing in periods of active rest? The problem is that you can maintain peak intensity for only a very short period of time; you must use intervals during which you train at peak intensity in short bursts, followed by moderately paced cardio (active rest), and then start all over again.

The Physiology of HIT

Similar to the engine of your car, which gradually cools down to a resting temperature at the end of a long journey, your body does the same after your exercise session. Once your workout is over, your body's metabolism can continue to burn more calories than when you are at complete rest. This physiological effect is called excess post-exercise oxygen consumption, also known as EPOC or oxygen debt. This relates to the amount of oxygen required to restore your body to homeostasis. The conditions inside the body must be well controlled if the body is to function effectively. Homeostasis is the maintenance of a constant internal environment.

Let us now take a look in more detail at how oxygen debt is achieved and how it is beneficial to us in terms of fat burning and weight loss.

As already discussed in section 5.3, the body is most efficient at producing ATP through aerobic metabolism (section 5.3.3). However, during the high-intensity phase, we are simply unable to supply oxygen at a rate that is fast enough to fuel our muscles. As a result, our anaerobic/lactate system (section 5.3.2) intervenes, using our intramuscular glycogen to assist in the provision of energy to the muscles for short bursts of activity. This type of training depletes the intramuscular glycogen quickly, within a couple of minutes.

Recovery should be active (e.g., walking between running intervals) to aid the return of blood to the liver, where glycogens are stored. The active recovery period allows aerobic glycolysis to produce and replace ATP in the involved muscles.

The by-product of anaerobic glycolysis is lactic acid, and as this builds up, you enter oxygen debt, and it is during the recovery phase that your heart and lungs work together to "pay back" this debt and break down the lactic acid. In other words, after completion of your intense training, your body has to repay that "borrowed energy" it owes to return your body to homeostasis. The more energy your body borrowed during the intense effort, the more oxygen it owes.

So why does it take more oxygen to recover? After exercise, there are other factors that cause an increase in oxygen consumption and repay the oxygen debt during the intense phase of your workout.

- During the recovery phase, breathing and heart rate are elevated (to remove carbon dioxide), and this requires more oxygen.
- Body temperature and metabolic rate are increased, again requiring more oxygen.
- Adrenaline and noradrenaline are increased, which in turn increases oxygen consumption.
- After exercise has stopped, extra oxygen is required to metabolize lactic acid; to replenish ATP, phosphocreatine, and glycogen; and to "pay back" any oxygen that has been borrowed from haemoglobin, myoglobin (an iron-containing substance, similar to haemoglobin, found in muscle fibres), air in the lungs, and the body's fluids. During this phase, the aerobic system is using oxygen to resynthesize intramuscular glycogen from lactate. In essence, the body is using lactic acid as a carbohydrate "middleman" to metabolize carbohydrates from your diet, without increasing insulin or stimulating fat synthesis. So lactic acid helps your body to burn more carbohydrates and ultimately more calories, assisting your weight-loss efforts.

After exercise has stopped, extra oxygen is required to metabolize lactic acid; to replenish ATP, phosphocreatine, and glycogen; and to "pay back" any oxygen that has been borrowed from haemoglobin, myoglobin (an iron-containing substance, similar to haemoglobin, found in muscle fibres), air in the lungs, and the body's fluids. During this phase, the aerobic system is using oxygen to resynthesize intramuscular glycogen from lactate. In essence, the body is using lactic acid as a carbohydrate "middleman" to metabolize carbohydrates from your diet, without increasing insulin or stimulating fat synthesis. So lactic acid helps your body to burn more carbohydrates and ultimately more calories, assisting your weight-loss efforts.

The Relevance of HIT to Fat Loss

The body expends approximately five calories of energy (a calorie is the amount of energy required to heat one litre of water by one degree centigrade) to consume one litre of oxygen. Therefore, increasing the amount of oxygen consumed both during and after a workout can increase the amount of net calories burned.

So, after an intense effort, you continue to breathe hard and your heart rate is elevated; your metabolism is operating at a higher rate to repay the oxygen it borrowed. The larger the oxygen debt created by your workout, the longer it will take to repay it, with the benefit of more calories being burned for a longer period of time after your training.

So What Is the Best Way to Create a Large Oxygen Debt?

It must be noted that the level of oxygen debt is influenced by the intensity of the exercise, not the duration. In order to create an oxygen debt, the effort has to be intense enough to switch over to "borrowed energy", or to an anaerobic mode. Therefore, pushing hard all the way before catching your breath is the best way of increasing oxygen debt, and this also increases the production of lactic acid. You should perform another intense exercise before the body has recovered to assist it in accumulating more lactic acid in the muscles. With enough intervals, you will cause a build-up of lactic acid and your body will in turn be able to burn more calories than normal after your workout has been completed. This is the rationale behind those fat-burning classes in which participants are requested to do different exercises one after another with little or no rest in between.

When the production of lactic acid exceeds the body's ability to disperse it, there will be a build-up of lactic acid—onset of blood lactate accumulation (OBLA). Targeted interval training improves this lactate tolerance. By performing high-intensity intervals, the body adapts and burns lactic acid (i.e., re-synthesizes intramuscular glycogen from lactate) more efficiently during exercise. As a result of this adaptation, you are able to exercise at a higher intensity for a longer period of time before fatigue or pain kicks in and slows you down.

How to Perform Effective Interval Training

An appropriate interval training routine should include just enough rest so that you are able to push hard for the next intense effort, and you should be breathing pretty hard when the whole series of intervals is complete.

Sprinting and resistance training are the best ways to accomplish this. Resistance training with compound exercises (exercises that involve more than one joint) for large muscle groups, such as those in the chest, back, glutes, and legs, places a greater demand on the involved muscles for ATP from the anaerobic glycolysis. Examples of such exercises include chest presses, pull-ups, deadlifts, and squats. (section 5.6). The increased need for anaerobic ATP also generates a greater demand on the aerobic system to replenish that ATP during the rest intervals (be sure to perform the next intense effort before your catch your breath) and the post-exercise recovery process. Heavy training loads or shorter recovery intervals increase the demand on the anaerobic energy pathways during exercise, yielding a greater oxygen debt during the post-exercise recovery period.

Combining intense efforts while already breathing hard is the best way to create maximum oxygen debt. This is one of the reasons why interval training is ideal for boosting the metabolism.

<u>Long-Term Benefits of Interval Training</u>

Interval training enables greater exposure to more intensive workouts without requiring an excessive amount of time exercising. Intensive repetition forces your body to respond by adapting to the new process; this is the principle of adaptation. The advantages include the following:

- Enhancement in lactic acid tolerance significantly improves athletic performance and well-being.
- Aerobic capacity is increased. Long-term adaptation includes an increase in capillarization, enabling more oxygen to be delivered to the muscles.
- Injuries associated with long-term repetitive exercises are significantly reduced, owing to a lack of overtraining or burnout.
- Overall cardiovascular fitness is improved.

- Insulin sensitivity is improved. Your muscles suck in glucose readily instead of the glucose going to your fat stores.

5.5.1 Types of Interval Training

Designing the correct interval training routine can be sophisticated or casual. Elite athletes may go to a <u>sports performance</u> laboratory to have their blood lactate and exercise metabolism tested to determine the optimum interval training routine. At the other end of the spectrum, casual "speed play" interval training (fartlek) can be adopted. You need to consult your exercise professional to select the most appropriate type of interval training to meet your goals.

There are different types of interval training; each is designed to target the energy systems mentioned above. Going into great detail about this is beyond the scope of this book, but table 5.5.1 illustrates the various forms of interval training that are designed to target the energy systems you wish to enhance.

Interval training programmes are now easily adapted to suit most sports. This is done by manipulating the intensity and duration of the work intervals, as well as the length of the rest periods, to create the desired adaptations.

<u>Training Variables</u>

- Duration (distance or time) of work interval
- Intensity (speed) of work interval
- Duration of rest or recovery interval
- Number of repetitions of each interval.

Energy System to Be Targeted	Time to Fatigue	Fuel Used	Predominant Muscle Fibre Type Involved	Target % Maximum Heart Rate	Work/Rest Ratio for Intervals	Recommended Number of Intervals Within the Session
ATP	3 seconds	ATP	Type 2b	NA	NA	NA
ATP–CP (Creatine Phosphate) (section 5.3.1)	10 seconds	Creatine phosphate	Type 2a and type 2b	90–100%	1:3 (e.g. 1 minute of exercise:3 minutes of active rest)	4-20
Lactic Acid (good for enhancing lactic tolerance*) (section 5.3.2)	60–90 seconds	Glycogen	Type 2a and type 1	70–90% (depending on fitness level)	1:3	4-5
Aerobic (sub-maximal) (section 5.3.3)	Long	Glycogen, fat and protein	Type 1	50%+	1:1	3-4

Table 5.5.1: Various Types of HITT to Target the Various Energy Systems

Safety Tips for Interval Training

Keep in mind that interval training is extremely demanding on the heart, lungs, and muscles, and it is important to seek medical clearance before you begin. You should also have a solid base of overall cardiovascular fitness before embarking on this type of training. You are advised to engage an exercise professional who will select the type of HIIT appropriate to your goals.

Interval training is an extremely beneficial form of exercise, but sometimes people push themselves too hard. This tends to result in sore muscles and joints, along with an increased likelihood of injury. It is important to consider the following precautions:

- Set a realistic training goal within your current fitness level.
- Warm up thoroughly prior to any exercise (section 5.4.1).
- Begin slowly and work towards longer intervals to obtain better results.
- Maintain a steady but challenging pace throughout the interval.
- To step up your fitness levels, increase the intensity or duration, but not both at the same time.
- Reduce your heart rate to 100–110 beats per minute during the rest interval.

Beginners should start with short intervals (under thirty seconds), fewer repeats, and more rest. Elite athletes can up the intensity, time, and frequency of their training. The added intensity of interval training requires your muscles and joints to be flexible, so you need to incorporate flexibility training into your fitness programme (section 4.3).

5.5.2 Cool-Down

After any exercise sessions, especially intense cardiovascular training, it is important to cool down to avoid blood pooling—the collection of blood in the lower limbs—and to help get blood back to the heart through the veins. Cool down by contracting muscles, which act as pumps to squeeze blood through the valves back to the heart in a process known as venous return.

During exercise, your muscles aid the return of the blood to the heart by contracting with more force around the blood vessels. This causes the blood to easily resist the forces of gravity and return quickly to the heart for reoxygenation and recirculation. When you stop exercising quickly, the muscles are no longer contracting against your veins; gravity causes the blood to pool in the lower extremities. When this occurs, you may feel faint or dizzy or experience a loss of consciousness.

<u>Teaching Points</u>

Cause your heart rate to rise to 50 per cent of MHR in the first minute, and then gradually lower it in the next four minutes (see diagram 5.5.2 below) to remove waste products and lactic acid.

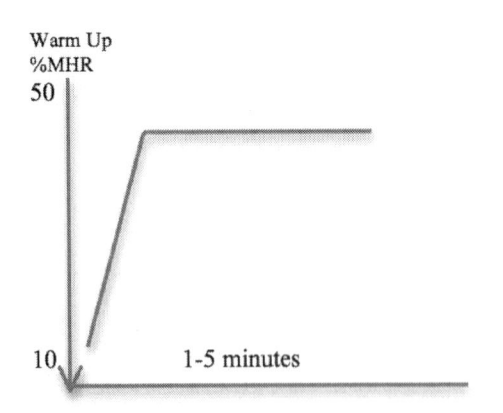

Diagram 5.5.2: Cool-Down

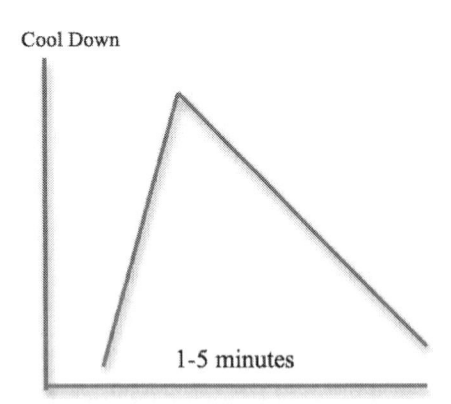

Summary

Please be reminded that losing weight and improving overall fitness is not just about exercising, it also involves other aspects of lifestyle, such as diet, work, rest, and management of stress. Before beginning any weight loss programme, it is important to ensure that it is safe. It is recommended that you first meet with a health professional who will advise you on your lower back condition and help to design an appropriate weight-loss programme for you.

Remember, obesity results when more calories are taken in than are burned by the body over a long period of time. Avoid consuming large, infrequent meals or lots of high-GI meals, as they will produce huge fluctuations in blood sugar and insulin. Insulin favours fat storage and suppresses the burning of fat as fuel.

If you are serious about weight management, you should avoid processed carbohydrates with a high glycaemic index. Furthermore, if you consistently eat more calories than you burn, you will not lose any body fat. Even if you exercise when your carbohydrate stores are depleted, as soon as you supply your body with more calories than you need, you start storing the excess as fat (triglycerides). In this case, you are essentially burning calories and storing fat. Even though you may be burning fat during exercise, the effect is only temporary. If you want to lose weight and body fat, the bottom line is that you must create a calorie deficit.

5.6 Exercises for Weight Loss: A Beginner's Guide to the Principle of Resistance Training

As previously discussed, one effective way of burning fat is to build more muscles using resistance training. This is because not only does muscle give your body its strength, shape and definition, it is also very metabolic. One kilogram of muscle can burn approximately one hundred calories per day, and the more muscle you have, the more calories you burn. As a result, building muscle through resistance training helps you to lose weight.

Before starting any exercise programme, you must work with your exercise professional to set a realistic and achievable goal by using the SMART principle:

- **S** = **Specific**: The goal must be clear and concise (e.g., "I want to lose ten kilograms.").
- **M** = **Measurable**: There must be a way of clearly comparing start and finish points. Some examples are your BMI, weight, and waist measurement. "Before and after" photos can also be a good motivational tool.
- **A** = **Achievable**: If the goals are too difficult to achieve or the timescale is too long, motivation will be lost (e.g., it is unrealistic and unsustainable to lose more than half a kilogram of weight per week).
- **R** = **Realistic**: The specific objective must be attainable within the set time frame.
- **T** = **Time-framed**: An exact and agreed amount of time must be established to focus efforts.

Warm-Ups

These warm-ups are similar to the cardiovascular session discussed in section 5.4.1. Apart from increasing your heart rate, warm-ups psychologically prepare you for the session. Most importantly, they mobilize your joints, allowing more synovial fluids to be released, lubricating your joints in preparation for the subsequent activities.

5.6.1 Dynamic Stretches

Dynamic stretches (static stretches should not be performed before resistance training, as they can impair your performance) should be done after your warm-up. "Dynamic" means that you are moving whilst you stretch. For a very long time in the past, static stretching, which requires holding a stretch for ten or more seconds while motionless, was advocated to be employed before exercise.

Your exercise professional will give you guidance on the type of dynamic stretch that you should perform prior to your resistance session. It is also advisable to perform a number of contractions using a lighter weight than prescribed for each resistance exercise in the programme.

Benefits of Dynamic Stretching

- It improves your range of motion.

- It activates muscles you will use during your workout. For example, a lunge with a twist is a dynamic stretch that engages your hips, legs, and core muscles. When you are actually exercising these muscles, they have already been involved during your dynamic stretch.

- Warming up in motion enhances muscular performance and power.

- It improves body awareness, because moving as you stretch challenges your balance and coordination—skills that could help your performance.

5.6.2 Repetitions (Reps)

The key to successful resistance training that fulfils your goal is first to establish the number of repetitions to be performed using a trial-and-error method. For example, if you decide to perform ten repetitions, you need to find a weight that you can lift successfully ten times only, but are unable to lift for an eleventh time. If you are able to perform more than ten repetitions, the weight is too light and you need to increase it. Conversely, if you are unable to perform the prescribed ten repetitions, you need to reduce the weight so you can lift it ten times but no more.

How do you decide upon the repetition range? It depends on what you wish to achieve. Common goals of resistance training include improving muscular endurance, size (hypertrophy), strength, and power (table 5.6.2.1).

RM	1	2	3	4	5	6	7	8	9	10	11	12	13	14	15	16	17	18	19	20
Strength																				
Power																				
Hypertrophy																				
Endurance																				

Table 5.6.2.1: The Resistance Exercise Continuum—Increased darkness in colour corresponds to increased adaptation for the relevant goal at the repetition maximum. RM = repetition maximum

The above guide highlights the intensity required to elicit specific gains. In simple terms, for strength gains (a heavy load with low repetitions), you are training your type 2b fibres (section 2.3), which acquire their energy through anaerobic glycolysis. At the other end of the spectrum, for muscular endurance (lighter loads with a higher number of repetitions, twelve to twenty-five), you are training your type 1 and type 2a fibres, which acquire their energy through aerobic glycolysis.

You are genetically programmed to have a certain percentage of each muscle fibre type. Those born with more type 2b fibres (e.g., those with a mesomorph body shape, section 5.6.9.2) are able to gain muscle size easier, and those with slower-twitch type 1 fibres (e.g., those with an ectomorph body shape, section 5.6.9.1) are more suited to endurance activities, such as marathons.

The amount of weight to be used can be based on a percentage of the individual's "one-repetition maximum" (1RM). 1RM is the maximum amount of weight that can be lifted once with good form. Likewise, 6RM is the maximum amount of weight that can be lifted six times.

An effective resistance training programme should reflect your needs. Table 5.6.2.2, below, outlines how to apply specific training principles to various training objectives.

Training Goal	Strength	Hypertrophy	Muscular Endurance
Intensity	High	Moderate	Low
Load as % of 1RM	>85%	67–85%	<67%
Repetitions	1–5	6–12	12+
Rest Time Between Sets	3–5 minutes	1–2 minutes	30–60 seconds
Sets Per Exercise	2–6	3–6	2–3
Frequency Per Muscle Group	1–2× per week	1–2× per week	2–3× per week

Table 5.6.2.2: Adapted from Baechle and Earle (2000)[11]

The concept of a progressive pyramid of training is outlined below (see diagram 5.6.2):

Beginners to resistance training should aim to build a foundation of muscular endurance and start with just two sessions per week. Intermediate or advanced users may have specific training goals that demand greater frequency and the application of more advanced training systems (section 5.6.8) with goals for muscular hypertrophy, strength, and power. These types of training should be attempted only once a solid foundation of technique, posture, basic cardiovascular fitness, and flexibility has been established.

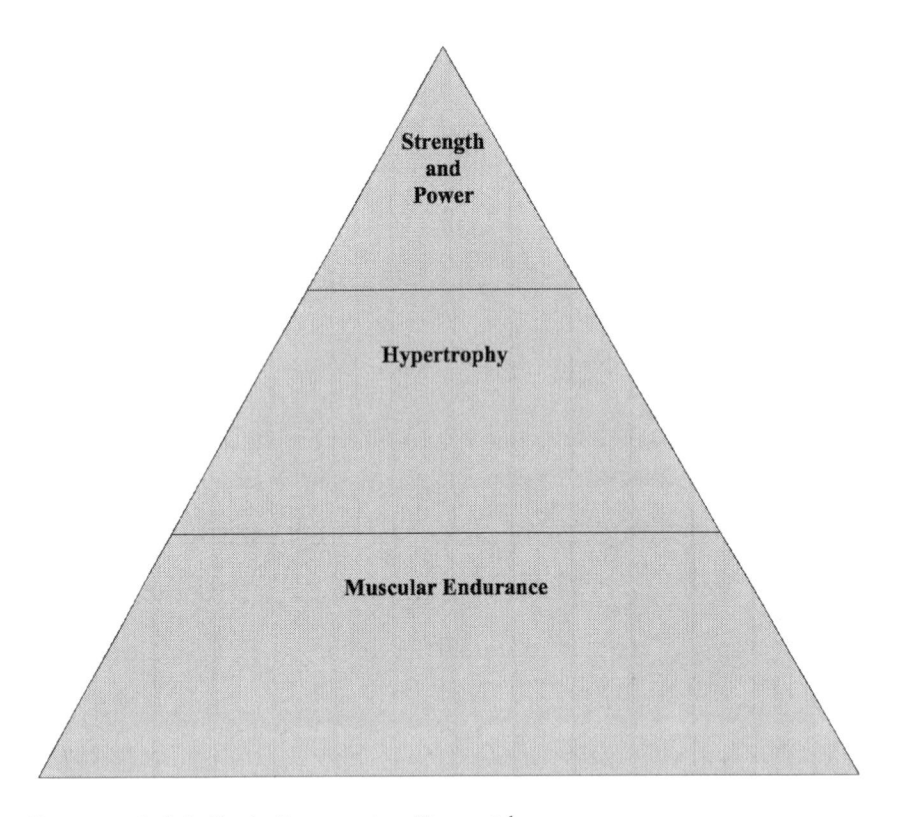

Diagram 5.6.2: Basic Progression Pyramid

There is scope for intensity progression within each of the three training objectives. For example, if you want to focus predominantly on muscular endurance, the guideline of twelve to twenty repetitions per set can be subdivided into smaller repetition ranges. Successive training phases (e.g., every fortnight) may progress from eighteen to twenty, fifteen to eighteen, and twelve to fifteen repetitions per set, with small increments in resistance (or weight) at each phase. The intensity increases, but repetitions performed still remain within the range for muscular endurance. Alternatively, you can amend other variables instead. You might increase the movement complexity from phase to phase while working with the same endurance repetition range. For instance, slowing down the speed of execution of movements, especially during the eccentric phase (section 5.6.7) will increase the intensity, as your muscles will be under tension for a longer period.

To achieve the desired results, it is important to focus on three interrelated elements of training:

1. **Training methods**

2. **Recovery:** It is important that you are aware that muscle growth does not actually take place whilst you are working out in the gym. This is because during resistance training exercise, muscle fibres are broken down, and in the days following the workout, the fibres repair and grow stronger to meet the demands that have been placed on them. Therefore rest days and ensuring you have the correct nutrition are as important as the exercise itself. You should have at least one rest day for each muscle group trained. Muscles can get stronger and bigger only when you stimulate them through hard exercise, helping them to recover with high-performance nutrition and giving them rest. The more intense you are, the more rest you need.

3. **Nutrition** (section 5.3.6).

5.6.3 Pros and Cons of Various Resistance Exercises (Machines or Free Weights)

As a general rule, if the purpose of performing these exercises is to lose weight and improve core stability to reduce back pain, using free weights is better than using machines, as this engages more of your core and stabilization musculatures (table 5.6.3 below).

	Advantages	**Disadvantages**
Machines	Machine exercises are easier to instruct and learn. The weight settings can be changed easily. The weight selected does not need to be calculated.	Machines work on a fixed plane of motion which is not functional (i.e., exercises on machines do not reflect actions in real life). They have a limited range of motion. They negate the use of core stabilizers. Use of machines results in a lack of synergist and fixator muscle engagement. Machines are more expensive than free weights.
Free Weights	Free-weight exercises can be performed anywhere. The equipment is less expensive. There is more functional engagement of synergist and fixator muscles.	Free-weight exercises are technique-sensitive and require more instruction than machine exercises.

Table 5.6.3: Pros and Cons of Different Types of Resistance Training

5.6.4 The Concept of "Balance Training"

An agonist (section 3.4), or prime mover, is a muscle that provides the major force needed to complete a movement. In a bicep curl, which produces flexion at the elbow, the biceps muscle is the agonist.

An antagonist is a muscle that opposes the agonist. During elbow flexion, where the biceps muscle is the agonist, the triceps are the antagonists; they typically relax so as not to impede the agonist.

Agonists and antagonists should be trained in the same session to avoid muscular imbalance. For instance, when you train your chest (pectorals) and shoulders (deltoids), you need to train the antagonists, the latissimi dorsi, as well. Likewise, when you train the quadriceps, you need to exercise the antagonists—the hamstring group of muscles. When you train your biceps, you need to train your triceps.

Excessive training of the chest while ignoring the back (the latissimi dorsi and the trapezii) leads to excessive tightening of the pectorals and a weak back, predisposing you to hyperkyphosis (section 6.2.2). This postural deviation can lead to back problems.

5.6.5 Effects of Resistance Training

"Adaptation" refers to how the body adjusts to repeated stress. For this to happen, there needs to be a systematic administration of a sufficient stimulus, followed by an adaptation by the individual involved, and then the introduction of a new, progressively greater, stimulus.

- **Strength adaptations:** The initial strength enhancement in the first couple of weeks of resistance training is primarily associated with neural adaptations, with the development of more efficient neural pathways by recruitment of more motor units (section 2.4). This adaptation will enable the muscle to generate more strength and force during muscle contractions. It is interesting to note that a beginner to resistance training is often able to recruit only a certain number of motor units in the beginning. This offers protection so that the muscles involved cannot develop too much force that could damage the muscle or connective tissues. As neuromuscular connections enhance progressively, the individual will gradually be able to recruit more motor units and produce more force and be able to lift heavier weights. Long-term changes in strength are more likely to be attributable to hypertrophy of the muscle fibres.

- **Muscle fibre adaptations:** The increase in size of a muscle is referred to as hypertrophy. Short-term hypertrophy is attributable to fluid accumulation, from blood plasma, in the intracellular and interstitial spaces of the muscle. Long-term hypertrophy is an increase in muscle size associated with long-term resistance training.

- **Bone tissue adaptations:** In response to the loading of the bone created by muscular contractions, bone tissue begins to remodel, resulting in a more rigid structure.

- **Heart rate adaptations:** Heart rate is acutely elevated immediately following a workout, but there appears to be a reduction in heart rate from resistance training, which is considered beneficial.

- **Body composition adaptations:** Resistance training can improve your body composition by increasing the fat-free mass and decreasing the percentage of body fat.

- **Glucose metabolism adaptations:** An important risk factor for cardiovascular disease and diabetes is glucose tolerance. High blood glucose and high insulin levels can also have a deleterious effect on hypertension and blood lipids. Strength and aerobic training improve glucose tolerance.

- **Blood pressure adaptations:** A short-term effect of resistance training is an increase in systolic blood pressure. Diastolic blood pressure may decrease slightly as a result of vasodilation. Heavy weight training will significantly increase both systolic and diastolic blood pressure. It is therefore important that you do not hold your breath when performing these activities in order to avoid the Valsalva effect. The increase in pressure within the thoracic cavity can impede the venous return of blood to your heart. Furthermore, the Valsalva effect can increase blood pressure and put you at risk of heart attack or stroke. You should breathe out during the concentric phase of muscle contraction and breathe in during the eccentric phase (section 5.6.7).

5.6.6 Sample Full-Body Resistance Training

As a general rule, perform compound exercises that involve multiple muscle groups (e.g., squats, deadlifts) before isolated exercises (e.g., bicep curls). Work on larger muscle groups (quadriceps, glutes and hamstrings, chest, back, and shoulders) before smaller muscle groups (biceps and triceps). See table 5.6.6 below.

Legs—Quadriceps Group Sample exercises • Deadlift • Leg press • Squat (body weight, jump squat, or with bar) • Leg extension	Legs—Hamstring Sample exercises • Leg curl • Lying leg curl • Floor glute-hamstring raise • Romanian deadlift with dumb-bells
Chest—Pectorals Sample exercises • Press-up • Chest bench press (barbell/dumb-bells) • Pec fly (cable/dumb-bells) • Chest machine	Back—Rhomboids and Latissimus Dorsi (6.4) Sample exercises • Seated row • Reverse body-weight row with Smith Machine or TRX • Single-arm row
Shoulder—Deltoids Sample exercises • Shoulder press with dumb-bells • Lateral raise • Front raise • Military press • Upright row • Various shoulder machines	Back—Trapezii and Latissimus Dorsi Sample exercises • Lat pull-down • Chin-up (assisted or body weight) • Isolated trapezius pull-down

Biceps	Triceps
Sample exercises	**Sample exercises**
• Dumbbell • Bar • EZ bar • Cable machine	• Triceps overhead extension • Triceps rope pull-down • Cable machine • Triceps kickback • Skull crusher

Table 5.6.6 Examples of a Full-Body Resistance Training Programme

There are many different exercises for each of the above groups of muscles, and only limited examples have been mentioned. When performing resistance training, you must brace your core (activate your transversus abdominis, Section 4.4.2.3) and keep your back straight so that your spine is protected.

The Need for Progression

Deconditioned novices have a large adaptation potential because they are starting from a point far below their genetic limit. Almost any programme will work for them, as they have a great adaptation potential and are unfamiliar with any exercise stimulus. They therefore tend to make rapid progress once exposed to the exercise stimulus. The rate of gain usually begins to slow down within a few weeks, and new stimuli need to be introduced. The same progression rules apply to almost everyone who participates in resistance training. Approximately every four to eight weeks, your exercise professional should modify the programme variables to generate a new exercise stimulus. If the workload of a training programme is not altered or progressed, individuals will not continue to adapt. Instead, once the body has become accustomed to the current workload, it will not attempt to adapt any further.

Prior to introducing you to the advanced techniques, it is worth making you aware that there are three types of muscle contractions.

5.6.7 Types of Muscle Contraction

<u>Isotonic contractions</u>

Isotonic contractions are those which cause the muscle to change length as it contracts and cause movement of a body part. There are two types of isotonic contraction:

Concentric

Concentric contractions are those that cause the muscle to shorten as it contracts. An example is flexing the elbow in a bicep curl or lifting a dumb-bell against gravity, causing a concentric contraction of the biceps brachii muscles.

Eccentric

Eccentric contractions occur when the muscle lengthens as it contracts. This is less common and usually involves the control or deceleration of a movement being initiated by the eccentric muscle's agonist. An example of this is when you extend your elbow at the end of a bicep curl, lowering the weight slowly in a controlled manner with gravity. Eccentric action thus prevents the weight from accelerating downward in an uncontrolled manner as a result of gravitational pull.

This type of contraction puts a lot of strain on the muscle and is commonly involved in injuries. Most muscle injuries are due to weakness in this type of muscle contraction.

It must be noted that gravity increases the eccentric demand on our muscles. We must therefore enhance our eccentric muscular strength accordingly; the eccentric action of training is just as important as the concentric action.

Isometric Contractions

Isometric contractions occur when there is no change in the length of the contracting muscle. This can happen when carrying an object in front of you as the weight of the object is pulling your arms down but your muscles are contracting to hold the object at the same level. Isometric actions dynamically stabilize the body. The plank (section 4.4.3) is an exercise to enhance the isometric strength of the transversus abdominis.

Effective resistance training must take into consideration the strength training of all three types of muscle contraction. Most gym-goers only concentrate on the concentric phase of their workout. Let us take the example of a chest bench press. The majority of people would concentrate on pushing up as much weight as possible, which involves concentric contraction of your pectorals, but let gravity take over by lowering the weight fairly quickly. You should lower the weight slowly and under control towards gravity, as this will improve the eccentric strength of your pectorals.

Holding the weight at the top momentarily before lowering (without locking your elbows) will strengthen the isometric strength of your pectorals.

Please consult your exercise professional for guidance.

5.6.8 Advanced Resistance Training Techniques

You must recognize that there is no such thing as a perfect single training routine or training system. Your body will adapt to any stimulus that is placed upon it relatively quickly. Your total volume of resistance training experience increases with each workout, you achieve gains in strength and muscular hypertrophy. It is common that with this transition our magnitude of increase in strength and muscle size diminishes, and eventually you will reach some form of plateau. It is therefore imperative that your exercise professional should look to modify the programme variables to generate a new exercise stimulus for you every four to eight weeks. You may therefore be introduced to the following advanced resistance techniques, which will enable you to grow more muscles; in turn, this will help you to burn more fat. This is because muscle tissue is metabolically active, and the more of it you have, the more calories you will burn—even at rest.

These following training techniques are not for beginners to resistance training and they should be performed only under the guidance of your exercise professional in order to maximize effectiveness and minimize the chance of you injuring yourself. No more than two or three of these advanced techniques should be employed in each training session.

Giant Set—The Big G

A giant set consists of four sets of four different exercises that work the same muscle group. The number of repetitions depends on what you are training for—power, strength, hypertrophy, or endurance (section 5.6.2). For example, a chest giant set might consist of ten reps on a flat bench press, ten reps of dumbbell flys, ten reps on a decline bench press, and ten reps of incline dumbbell presses. You can adapt the giant set to other muscle groups (i.e., back, legs, arms etc.), and you can create any combination of four corresponding exercises.

When performing a giant set, quickly move from exercise to exercise. Your rest period should not exceed ten seconds. You need to push yourself hard to generate more muscle hypertrophy. When you have finished a giant set of the four exercises, rest for two minutes and then perform two more giant sets. When you are done, you will have performed twelve sets of exercises.

Besides providing amazing strength benefits, giant sets elevate your metabolism. Since there is very little time for rest, giant sets provide good cardiovascular benefits, and essentially this is a type of high-intensity interval training (section 5.5). Therefore, giant sets are extremely effective at building muscle and burning fat.

Tri-Set

A tri-set involves three exercises back to back, similar to giant sets but only three exercises for the same muscle group are performed rather than four. For instance, shoulder press (compound exercise for the deltoids), shoulder lateral raise (isolation exercise for the lateral deltoid), and front raise (isolation exercise for the anterior deltoid).

Pre-Exhaustion Training (A Type of Superset Training)

Pre-exhaust a given muscle with an isolation exercise (an exercise used to tackle one specific muscle group or joint in isolation), and then finish off with a compound exercise (an exercise that requires more than one joint and more than one muscle group). For example, perform leg extensions (an isolation exercise for the quadriceps) before squats (a compound exercise involving more than one muscle group). The theory is that fatiguing a muscle with an isolation exercise before a compound exercise will lead to greater muscle recruitment.

However, it is worth noting that pre-exhaustion exercises can affect your form, and as a result, you may be more prone to injury when employing this type of training. Post-exhaustion training is therefore safer.

Post-Exhaustion Training (Compound First, Then Isolation Exercise)

Similar to pre-exhaustion training, but a compound exercise is performed first, and then an isolation exercise; e.g., a bench chest press and then a chest fly.

Super Slow: Ten Seconds Concentric and Ten Seconds Eccentric (Same Reps)

The super-slow technique involves moving very slowly through repetitions for both the lifting (concentric phase) and lowering movements (eccentric phase) of each exercise. A ten-second count is used. There is no help from momentum, and there's no rest in between each repetition. This type of training is very intense on the body, as each repetition takes a total of twenty seconds to complete; it may take a week for the muscles to fully repair and rebuild.

Because the movements are so slow, this technique is also a great way to reduce the risk of injury and improve the eccentric strength of your muscles (section 5.6.7).

Forced Reps

Forced reps are an effective strength-training strategy to increase muscle mass, but they need to be done with the assistance of an exercise partner. For instance, when you are performing your final set of bench chest presses, and are approaching **muscle failure** (the point of being unable to finish a repetition, not when you cannot do an additional repetition; you literally attempt the repetition but fail to complete it), your partner grabs the bar and instructs you to continue. By assisting the movement, he is lifting some of the weight for you and so you continue to push. As your muscles continue to reach fatigue, your partner provides a heavier and heavier spot, and so you continue until he is doing most of the work.

The idea behind forced sets is similar to that of drop sets. By lightening the weight, you are able to move past your initial muscle failure and eventually approach absolute muscle failure. Forced sets tear deep into muscle tissue and result in increased muscle growth. However, they are extremely taxing and should not be used for each set. So while they are a great muscle building technique, use them sparingly—say, no more than once every fortnight.

Negative Sets, Also Known as Eccentric Training

Employing negative sets is a powerful technique for rapid strength gains, and it is effective at breaking through stubborn plateaus. Negative training involves loading the resistance beyond your maximum and effectively training only the eccentric movement (section 5.6.7). You will need the help of a spotter for the concentric portion.

If you are performing negative sets on a bench press, it's generally recommended that negatives should be started at 105 per cent of your one-rep max (one-repetition maximum - i.e., the amount of weight you could press if you were doing just one repetition). Assuming that your one-rep max is 100 kilograms, you would load the bench press with 105 kilograms of weight.

Your partner stands behind the bench and provides you with the required assistance. When lowering the bar towards your chest (eccentric phase), take twice as much time as usual. Once the bar touches your chest, your partner will help you to lift the bar and return it to the starting position. Repeat the whole process again.

Negative sets are very tough on your muscle fibres, and there is no need to do more than three negative sets. You need to give you muscles adequate recovery time after your workout.

Perform negative sets on those exercises that can be easily and effectively spotted, such as the bench press or barbell bicep curls.

Negative sets should not be the backbone of your workout routine, because they ignore concentric training. Instead, use negative sets as a tool for breaking through plateaus or to spice up your routine.

Superset

A superset is the performance of two exercises back-to-back without rest. Supersets can pair targeted muscle groups, as listed below.

> *Agonist/agonist* – for example, a hammer curl and a bicep curl. Supersets performed on the same muscle group will mean hitting that muscle harder; you will make some impressive strength gains, and it is also an effective way of breaking through that stubborn plateau.
>
> *Agonist/antagonist* – supersets performed on the opposing muscle groups; for example, a bicep curl and a triceps extension.
>
> *Agonist/synergist* – for example, a bench press/triceps pull-down.
>
> The advantage of using supersets to train different muscle groups—for example, chest and back workouts (agonist/

antagonist)—is that it allows you to do more in less time by cutting out extra rest periods. Instead of sitting around for sixty seconds during a rest period, you are able to go on to another exercise for a different muscle group. You will still get the recovery you need whilst working another muscle group in the meantime.

Drop Set / Strip set

Drop sets may be one of the most effective muscle-building techniques. You perform a set of any exercise to failure (or just short of failure) for between eight and twelve reps, and then drop some weight (usually 15 per cent) and continue for additional repetitions with the reduced resistance. Once failure has again been reached, additional resistance is dropped, and so on.

Pyramid sets

Ascending Pyramid

In an ascending pyramid set, the first set of an exercise is performed at a low weight for a high number of repetitions. The resistance (or weight) in each subsequent set is increased until a final set of a heavy weight and very few reps is achieved. For people just starting to exercise, they might try three sets of increasingly heavy weights and decreasing repetitions. For those with more experience, five sets of twelve, ten, eight, six, and then four repetitions can be achieved.

>Example:
>Twelve reps—10 kg
>Ten reps—15 kg
>Eight reps—20 kg
>Six reps—25 kg

Descending Pyramid

For a descending pyramid set, lower the amount of resistance once you have reached your maximum, and eventually return to your starting weight.

> Example:
> Six reps—25 kg
> Eight reps—20 kg
> Ten reps—15 kg
> Twelve reps—10 kg

Full Pyramid

To perform a full pyramid set, start with an ascending pyramid set and follow with a descending pyramid set.

Pyramid sets are ideal for building muscle mass and it is recommended that you incorporate pyramid sets for those muscle groups that you would like to increase in size.

Matrix 21s

The technique known as matrix 21s has three phases of movement and twenty-one repetitions. It is usually used for bicep curls, and the action is split into three phases.

The matrix system is based on a patterned series of partial movements designed to activate muscle fibres at multiple points not otherwise worked very effectively during conventional exercise. This exploits the body's potential to produce gains in muscle size and strength much faster than with conventional weight training.

1. Perform seven repetitions of top-range partial bicep curls where you only lower the bar halfway.

2. Then, perform seven repetitions of low-range partial curls, stopping halfway up.

3. Finish with seven repetitions with a full range of motion.

Because matrix training does not rely on heavy weights to achieve maximal intensity, the risk of muscle strain and injury is greatly reduced. For this reason, the matrix system is ideally suited to a wide range of users, including those with injuries that would normally prevent them from weight training.

5.6.9 How Body Type Influences the Response to Training and Weight Loss

Body type (see diagram 5.6.9 below) influences how you respond to training, as well as the effectiveness of your weight-loss programme. Therefore, understanding your body type is important in making your training and weight loss effective, because different body types require different training stimuli and diet plans.

5.6.9.1 Ectomorph

An ectomorph is a typical skinny person with a light build, small joints, lean muscle and long, thin limbs. Their shoulders tend to be thin and narrow, and their chests are flat. They find it hard to gain weight and tend to have a fast metabolism, which burns calories very quickly. They therefore need a huge amount of calories in order to gain weight. Workouts should be short and intense, focusing on big muscle groups. Ectomorphs should eat before bedtime to prevent muscle catabolism during the night. Generally, ectomorphs can lose fat very easily, which makes cutting back to lean muscle easier for them.

James Tang

Body types

Ectomorph   Mesomorph   Endomorph

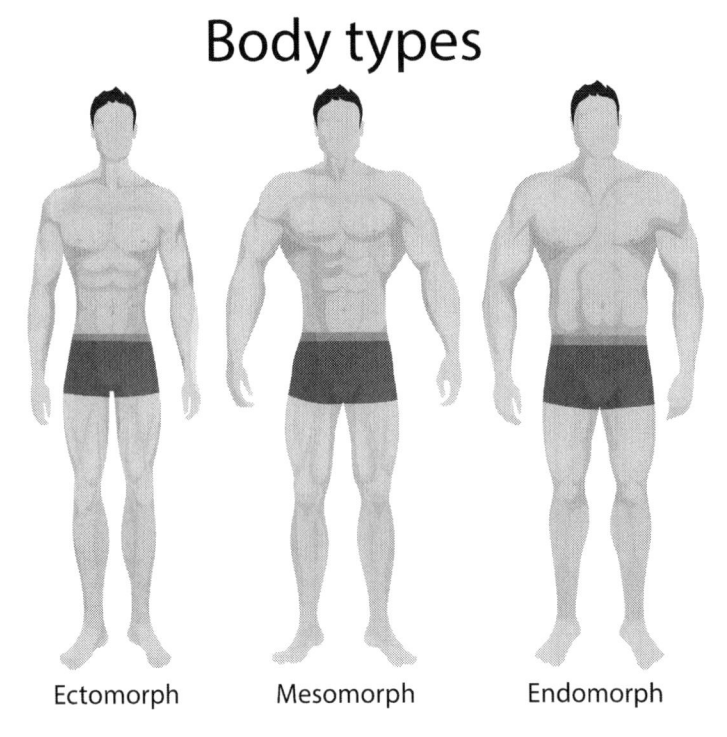

Diagram 5.6.9: Body Types

5.6.9.2 Mesomorph

A mesomorph has a large bone structure, large muscles, and a naturally athletic physique. They have the best body type for bodybuilding. They find it quite easy to gain and lose weight, and are naturally strong, which is perfect for building muscles. They respond the best to weight training, as gains are usually seen very rapidly, especially for beginners. However, they gain fat more easily than ectomorphs, and they must watch their calorie intake. Usually, a combination of weight training and cardio works best for mesomorphs.

5.6.9.3 Endomorph

The endomorph body type is solid and generally soft with a round physique, but poor muscle definition. Endomorphs have a slow metabolism, gain fat easily, and find it hard to lose fat. They are usually of shorter build with thick arms and legs. Endomorphs find that they are naturally strong in leg exercises, such as the squat.

It is very easy for endomorphs to gain weight but, unfortunately, a large portion of this weight is fat not muscle. In order to minimize fat gain, endomorphs must always do cardio training as well as weights.

A Combination of Body Types

Given this information, you should be able to identify your body type; it is quite possible that you are a combination of all three. Irrespective of your body type, you can still build a big, ripped, muscular physique, and even the skinniest person can bulk up. Yes, it may be harder, but if you are willing to put in the hard work, it can be done.

Conclusion

Please remember that after every training session, you need to cool down (section 5.5.2) and perform static stretches (section 4.3) and, preferably, some core stability exercises (section 4.5.1).

As you may appreciate, the theories behind resistance training are complex, sometimes contradictory and constantly changing. So, with regard to obesity and lower back pain, only a simplistic overview of training involving weights has been discussed here. If you have medical conditions, such as cardiovascular, pulmonary, or metabolic disease, or other conditions that may be aggravated by exercise (e.g., arthritis), please seek medical clearance prior to embarking on a programme of exercises.

It is imperative that you consult an exercise professional who can devise the most appropriate diet plan and exercise programme for you, based on the FITT principle and according to your SMART goals.

FITT is an acronym:

> **F = frequency** (how frequently you participate in each particular exercise).
> **I = intensity** (the weight you use, the repetitions and the number of sets).
> **T = time** (rest time between each set and between sessions).
> **T = type of exercise** (equipment used, free weights, machines, kettlebells, bodyweight etc.).

Your exercise professional does not only supervise your technique or form, he or she can monitor your progress by making variations to your training routines. As you can see, there are so many interacting variables that can affect the results of your training. Apart from the types of exercise that you do, weight that you lift, techniques that you adopt, number of repetitions, number of sets, and resting time between sets, other variables include:

- **Movement speed** – the pace of weightlifting can significantly affect the effectiveness of the workout (e.g., pushing against gravity at a fast pace is much easier than performing the same action slowly in a controlled movement, because your muscles will be under tension for a lot longer with the second approach).

- **Stable to unstable exercise positions** – overall stability is important when you train for core stability (section 4.5.1).

CHAPTER 6

Postural Dysfunction

6.1 Introduction to Posture

<u>What Is Posture?</u>

On any given day, we all spend a lot of time in certain positions (e.g., sitting in a chair at work). The term "posture" typically refers to how the body positions itself as a whole; "good" posture indicates a certain positioning in which our spinal curves remain neutral, not bent forward, backward, or sideways. It is the state of muscular and skeletal balance that protects the supporting structures of the body against injury or progressive deformity during rest or action. If one of your postures puts your spine out of its natural alignment, your muscles will adapt and become unbalanced. This is called a postural dysfunction.

As explained in section 3.2.1, one of the most common causes of lower back pain is a muscle imbalance which renders the muscle involved weak and dysfunctional, and the most common cause of muscle imbalance is poor posture. It must be emphasized that not everyone with postural deviation will exhibit pain symptoms. We should, however, not be complacent because it is most likely that we have harboured latent trigger points (section 4.2.4.5) in our muscles and these can easily be activated, with back pain being the result.

Neutral Spine

The spine has four natural curves in the saggital plane (when viewed from the side, see diagram 6.1.1), and they are essential for shock absorption. These curves are as follows:

1. Cervical lordosis—formed from seven cervical vertebrae.
2. Thoracic kyphosis—found in the chest, thorax, and the ribs; formed from twelve vertebrae.
3. Lumbar lordosis—found in the lower back, the lumbar region; formed from five vertebrae.
4. Sacral kyphosis—formed from two sets of fused bones: the sacrum (comprising five fused bones to make one unit) at the base of the spine, and the coccyx (comprising four fused bones and also known as the tail bone)

Each section of the spine forms a curve with the segment below being a curve in the opposite direction to the one above. So, the cervical curve is an anterior curve with the thorax being a posterior curve; the lumbar is anterior with the sacral/coccyx curve being posterior. These curves are interdependent; a change in one curve will result in a change in the curve above or below it.

In a neutral position, the spine is supported mostly by the bony structures of the vertebrae resting on top of one another. When these curves become either exaggerated or flattened, the spine increasingly relies on muscles, ligaments, and soft tissues to maintain an upright position, causing tension in these structures, with the consequential formation of adhesion and trigger points (section 4.2.4). Over time, this can even lead to spinal disc injury. In fact, Travell and Simons[12] suggested that trigger points may be the most common cause of herniated discs, because shortening or tightening the muscles could be the main source of disc compression and spinal nerve impingement.

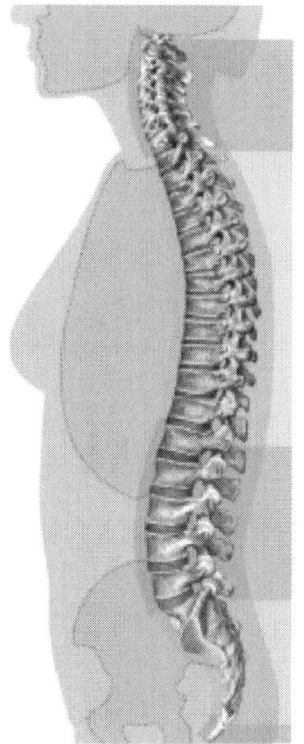

Cervical Lordosis

Thoracic Kyphosis

Lumbar Lordosis

Sacral Kyphosis

Diagram 6.1.1: Natural Spinal Curvatures

Postural Assessment

How do we know if our posture is ideal? Postural assessment is performed to identify any deviation from a neutral posture so that we can highlight any areas of dysfunction. A basic postural assessment can be done either statically or dynamically.

We need to check if the shoulders are at the same level and whether there is any anterior or posterior pelvic tilt etc. When in a neutral position, the anterior superior iliac spine (ASIS, a projection at the anterior end of the iliac crest) is slighter lower than the posterior superior iliac spine (PSIS, a projection at the posterior end of the iliac crest). A spine is hyperlordotic when PSIS is more than two centimetres above ASIS. Are your feet excessively pronated (flat feet, see chapter 7)? You may not be suffering from any musculoskeletal symptoms despite having postural deviations, but prevention is better than cure. If you identify your postural deviation early, you can consciously correct it to avoid future problems relating to muscle imbalances.

There should be a straight vertical line joining these points of reference in an ideal posture (see diagram 6.1.2 below):

- The ear lobe
- The centre of the shoulder (acromion process)
- The elbow
- The centre of the hip (greater trochanter)
- A point slightly anterior to the midline of the knee
- A point slightly anterior to the lateral malleolus.

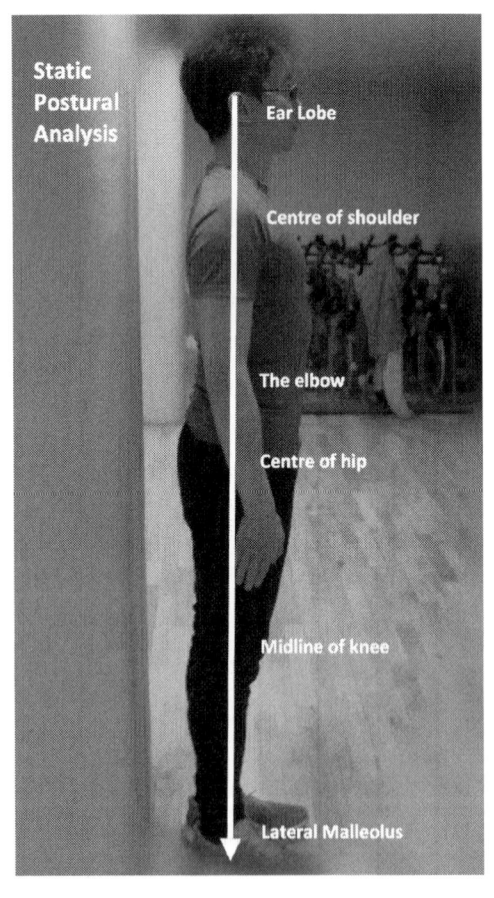

Diagram 6.1.2: Static Postural Analysis

Poor posture can lead to misalignment of the pelvis, causing imbalances of muscles attached to the lumbo-pelvic-hip complex. Common types of misaligned pelvis include the following:

- Anterior pelvic tilt
- Posterior pelvic tilt
- Twisted pelvis - such pelvic asymmetry creates stress at the sacroiliac (SI) joints (chapter 8). Pelvic rotation occurs at the sacroiliac joints, which facilitate gait dynamics. Postural asymmetry of the pelvis is common, and this leads to compensatory movement elsewhere and imbalances of the muscles that are attached to the lumbo-pelvic-hip complex in both static and dynamic postures.

Adverse Effects of Postural Deviations

- Muscle imbalances (section 3.2)
- Synergistic dominance (section 3.6)
- Increased risk of injury (section 6.2.8) and development of trigger points (section 4.2.4)
- Increased risk of aches and pains
- Increased stress on the joints
- Altered function of associated body systems (section 6.2.2).

6.2 Common Postural Deviations

6.2.1 Hyperlordosis

There is a natural lordotic curve, but if it is excessive, you have hyperextension (excessive backwards bending) of your spine, and the front of your pelvis will be tilted forward (anterior pelvic tilt) and downward.

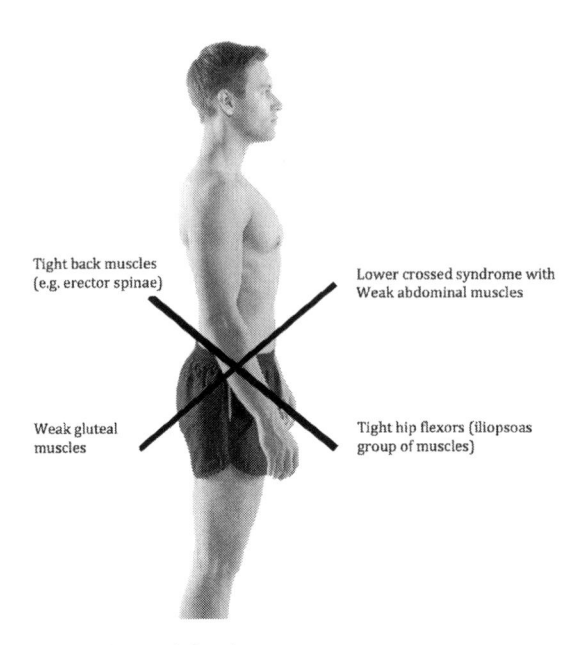

Diagram 6.2.1: Lower Crossed Syndrome

Hyperlordosis is usually due to a muscular imbalance causing lower crossed syndrome (see diagram 6.2.1 above). Certain muscles (typically postural muscles) are shortened in response to stress, such as prolonged sitting, and they in turn inhibit their antagonists on the other side of the joint as a result of reciprocal inhibition (section 3.5). The iliopsoas (hip flexors), the lumbar erector spinae (section 4.2.6.4), and the quadratus lumborum (section 4.2.6.5) are often tight. These in turn then inhibit or weaken the abdominal muscles, including the transversus abdominis (section 4.4.2.3) and the gluteus maximus (section 4.4.2.1).

The iliopsoas is an important culprit in hyperlordosis, since as well as tilting the pelvis anteriorly, it also inhibits the gluteus maximus, preventing it from resisting the forward tilting of the pelvis. Inhibition of the glutes can cause other muscles to overwork as a result of synergistic dominance (section 3.6) resulting in the formation of trigger points (section 4.2.4) in these synergist muscles, a common cause of lower back pain.

Pain can also arise directly as a result of hyperlordosis due to the increased lumbar curve causing the facet joints of the lumbar vertebrae to remain closed during functional movements. This leads them to become irritated, causing pain through the joints' nociceptors (pain receptors). In addition, the nerve roots that pass through the affected vertebral segment may be compressed by the excessive lumbar hyperextension. This type of nerve pain can create symptoms of sciatica (section 4.3.2.5).

Apart from prolonged sitting, other causes of lower crossed syndrome are as follows:

- Abdominal obesity and pregnancy, which shift the centre of gravity forward owing to the excess weight of the abdomen.
- Prolonged standing with a weak abdominal core - with the abdominal muscles being weak, they are unable to resist the downward pull by the iliopsoas. Abdominal muscles can be weak because of either surgery or underuse (section 3.3).
- The wearing of high heels – when you wear high heels, if there is no compensation in your body, your torso will lean forward as a result of the extra height from the shoes. As a consequence, the body compensates for this forward angle by hperextending the spine, leading to hyperlordosis, and an anterior tilting of the pelvis.

Anterior pelvic tilt is a very common form of postural deviation—much more common than you might think. You can check whether you have this postural deviation by standing sideways in front of a mirror. Watch to see if your pelvis tilts upwards when you simultaneously activate your TvA (section 4.4.2.3) and glutes (section 4.4.2.1). If so, you have a habitual anterior pelvic tilt. Since the lower crossed syndrome is due to weakness of the glutes and abdominal muscles; activating these muscles can effectively reverse the anterior tilting of the pelvis and return it to its "normal" position (see corrective exercises for hyperlordosis in section 6.3). The lesson that we learn here is that once we have noticed our postural problems, we need to consciously correct them in our everyday routine. Although this may feel awkward in the beginning, it is definitely worthwhile for the prevention of muscle imbalances and back pain.

6.2.2 Hyperkyphosis

Hyperkyphosis is characterized by an excessive thoracic spinal flexion (forward bending of the spine), typically associated with protracted shoulders, forward head posture, and posterior tilting of the pelvis, leading to imbalances of muscles that are attached to the lumbo-pelvic-hip complex.

Causes of hyperkyphosis are as follows:

- Postural/musculoskeletal hyperkyphosis: This is the most common form of hyperkyphosis, typically a result of poor posture with no vertebral deformities. This type of postural dysfunction is particularly prevalent in those who work in offices and spend a lot of time sitting at the desk, hunching their back whilst working on their computers. As well as being due to poor postural habits, postural hyperkyphosis is commonly noticeable in the gym in those who overtrain their pectorals but routinely neglect to train the antagonist, the latissimus dorsi. The stronger pectorals pull the shoulder girdle out of position (rounded shoulders) and their whole body will end up making adjustments to compensate, ultimately leading to hyperkyphosis.
- Scheuermann's disease: This is the juvenile form of hyperkyphosis.
- Congenital hyperkyphosis: This is a bone defect that can be detected at birth.
- Age-related hyperkyphosis: A kyphosis angle that increases with age, sometimes referred to as dowager's hump, and this may develop from either muscle weakness or degenerative disc diseases.
- Neurological hyperkyphosis: This can be the result of the paralysis of the abdominal muscles.

Only postural hyperkyphosis will be considered in this book.

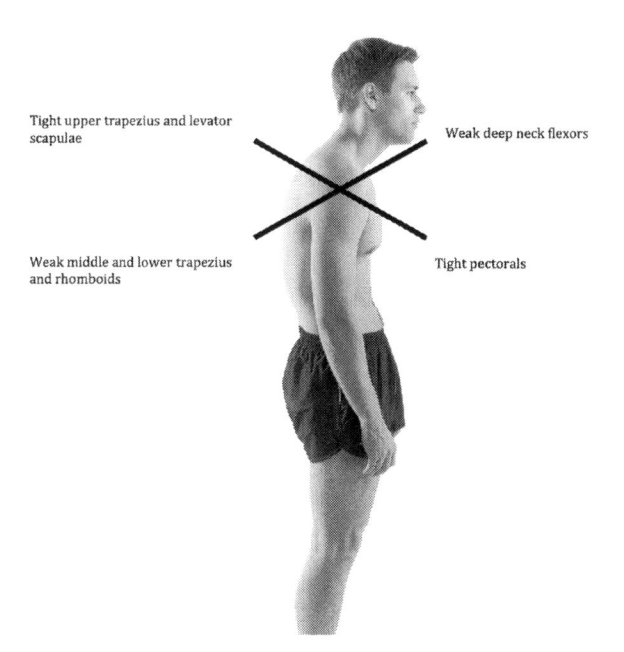

A Practical Guide to the Self-Management of Lower Back Pain

Diagram 6.2.2: Hyperkyphosis

Characteristics of Hyperkyphosis

- **Muscle imbalances**: Hyperkyphosis is also known as upper crossed syndrome and is characterized by tight upper trapezius, levator scapulae, and pectorals (chest muscles), along with protracted shoulders, weak deep neck flexors, rhomboids, and middle and lower trapezius etc. Apart from lower back pain due to posterior pelvic tilt, pain is often reported in the neck, shoulder, chest, and thoracic spine.
- "Rounded" shoulders - this condition predisposes you to impingement of the supraspinatus (one of the four rotator cuff muscles) tendon due to reduction of the subacromial space.
- Posteriorly tilted pelvis - this affects the length-tension relationship (section 2.6) of the muscles that are attached to the lumbo-pelvic-hip complex (e.g., lengthening of back muscles, such as the erector spinae group, and tightening of the abdominal muscles, such as the rectus abdominis, leading to muscle dysfunction and lower back pain).

- **Forward head posture**: Maintaining the natural cervical (neck) lordosis is important, but the author has observed that forward head posture is prevalent amongst the general population. In fact, forward head posture, although a common feature of those with hyperkyphosis, can occur independently. Do you notice when you drive that you often comfortably rest your body and shoulders on the seat but your head is usually not on the headrest? If so, this means that your head is being forwardly translated and you are adopting a forward head posture when you drive, even though you may not be aware of this. You can test if you have a habitual forward head posture by aligning your body with your back against the wall; do you need to move your head back consciously for it to touch the wall? If so, you adopt a habitual forward head posture. Spending a prolonged period of time in this posture can predispose you to upper shoulder and neck pain, because as previously mentioned, forward head posture is commonly associated with upper crossed postural distortion syndrome.

By holding the head in an unbalanced forward position, the cervical vertebrae can no longer adequately support the spine, and the muscles of the neck and upper shoulder must contract constantly in order to support the weight of the head in the forward position, resulting in tension neck syndrome, which is characterized by headaches and chronic pain in the neck and shoulder.

Forward head posture is a result of imbalances between the muscles that support and move the neck, shoulders, and head. The weight of the head is approximately 10 per cent of total body weight. The muscles at the back of the neck (neck extensors) are activated constantly to support the weight of the head in a forward position. Those muscles at the front of the neck that are responsible for it flexing and forward bending (the deep neck flexors) may become weakened and inhibited through reciprocal inhibition (section 3.5), resulting in an extended cervical spine (with the head bending backwards) with a shortened/tightened upper trapezius, sternocleidomastoid (SCM), and anterior scalene muscles. Furthermore, a forward head posture accentuates the anterior shear force at the cervical spine, and this posture results in the levator scapulae contracting constantly to dynamically minimize this force.

Forward head posture is also harmful to the intervertebral discs, possibly causing disc degeneration and herniation. This situation is similar to a posture in which the head is held to one side (lateral flexion of the neck); this is a common issue even though people are often unaware of it.

Diagnosis of Forward Head Posture

The powerful sternocleidomastoid muscles can easily be observed through the skin and can therefore serve as an indicator of a forward head posture. The greater the verticality of the sternocleidomastoid muscles when the neck is viewed from the side, the greater the likelihood that a forward head posture is present. This is because bilateral contraction of these muscles is responsible for the head being translated forward.

Trigger Points in the Neck and Shoulder

It is perhaps confusing, but the majority of neck pain is caused by trigger points in the upper back (e.g., the trapezius) and interscapular muscles (e.g., the rhomboids). Trigger points in the neck typically refer pain to the head, causing headaches. For example, tightness of the sternocleidomastoid does not cause pain in the muscle itself; frontal headaches are characteristic of sternocleidomastoid trigger points. These trigger points can even initiate an autonomic eye response, such as lachrymation (tearing) or visual disturbance. Trigger points in the scalene muscles of the neck refer pain to the back, shoulders, and arms. Generally speaking, trigger points tend to refer pain to a different location, and performing self-myofascial release (SMR) on the areas where pain is felt may not provide relief (section 4.2.4).

It is beyond the scope of this book to go into the details of SMR for the neck. Please be reminded that although aches and pains from trigger points are common, there can sometimes be an underlying pathology. It is always advisable to seek a proper diagnosis if you suffer from neck or back pain.

Effects of Hyperkyphosis on the Functioning of the Body

Besides back, shoulder and neck pain, hyperkyphosis may affect the functioning of the body because if the condition is not treated and the spinal curve continues to worsen over time, it may affect your ability to breathe. This happens because such severe spinal deformities inevitably end up warping the ribcage, leaving less room for your lungs to inflate, resulting in compromised breathing.

Severe hyperkyphosis can also impact your digestive system. This may be due to the internal organs being squashed together, potentially obstructing the passage of food through the intestines.

Furthermore, severe hyperkyphosis can result in nerve impingement and, depending on the location of compression, symptoms can range from persistent aches/pains, numbness or tingling sensations and weakness of certain body parts, to loss of bladder/bowel control.

Although these consequences of hyperkyphosis are rare, it is imperative that you seek appropriate advice once you have been identified as having a hyperkyphotic posture so as to prevent progression of the condition, and minimize the impact on your general health.

6.2.3 Scoliosis

Scoliosis is a condition in which the spine bends abnormally to the side, either to the right or left. In around eight out of every ten cases, the cause of scoliosis is not established, and this is known as idiopathic scoliosis. In recent years, scoliosis has become more common as a result of the modern lifestyles. People who routinely carry heavy bags on one side or who spend a lot of time resting a telephone on one shoulder may develop scoliosis. Improper work ergonomics may also lead to scoliosis; for instance, spending a prolonged period with your torso in a twisted position (e.g., in an attempt to work on a computer placed on a table to one side).

Generally speaking, there are three treatment options for scoliosis, depending upon the severity of the condition: observation, bracing, and surgery. Certain exercises may be prescribed by your doctor or physiotherapist, but they are not a means of treatment. Treatment for moderate to severe scoliosis will most likely involve surgery.

Back pain is the primary symptom of scoliosis, especially in lumbar scoliosis, due to imbalances of the muscles to the right and left side of the spinal curvature. Mild scoliosis that is not conspicuous will usually not require significant medical intervention. Scoliosis is considered to be mild if the deviation of the spinal curvature is less than 20 degrees. This type of scoliosis is the most responsive to corrective exercises.

An in-depth analysis of scoliosis and the associated corrective exercises is beyond the scope of this book as this condition must be treated by an appropriate professional. It is therefore important to seek medical advice before engaging in corrective exercises for scoliosis. This will ensure that you will not be harming your skeletal system by performing these activities.

Other Variations of the Above Three Major Postural Deviations

6.2.4 Sway Back Posture

The sway back posture is a posture in which the pelvis is pushed in front of the centre of gravity. This causes a chain reaction in the posture as the body attempts to compensate for the shift in alignment. Sway back posture is characterized by the following:

- The hip swaying forward and the pelvis being pushed forward in front of the centre of gravity
- The thorax being pushed back
- Posterior pelvic tilt
- Flat, lower lumbar lordosis.

6.2.5 Military Posture

This type of posture is often mistaken as a neutral posture and is typified by the chest being pushed forward and up. It is commonly associated with hyperlordosis and an anterior pelvic tilt.

6.2.6 Slumped Posture

This is a combination of hyperkyphosis (section 6.2.2) and hyperlordosis (section 6.2.1)

6.2.7 Flat-Back Posture

As the name implies, there is a reduction or elimination of the normal lumbar spinal curvature in this posture, typically resulting in a posterior pelvic tilt. Due to the reduction of the natural lumbar lordosis, it is commonly compensated for by a forward head posture.

6.2.8 Cumulative Injury Cycle (Diagram 6.2.8)

Over a long term, if we do not correct our postural deviations, there will be consequences. Lower back, neck, shoulder, hip and knee pain are often results of bad posture. You must therefore recognize your postural deviations and attend to them as much as possible in order to avoid these injuries.

As mentioned in section 2.8, the human movement system is an integrated and multidimensional system. If one component of the kinetic chain (muscular, skeletal, and nervous systems) is out of alignment, patterns of tissue overload and dysfunction will follow. This misalignment, if left uncorrected, will result in a vicious circle of injury, which is known as the cumulative injury cycle.[13] The cycle starts with tissue trauma, leading to inflammation, which activates your body's pain receptors. This causes an increase in muscle tension at the site of trauma, causing your muscle spindles (which are sensitive to the change in length and the rate of the change in length) to spasm, resulting in the formation of trigger points (section 4.2.4) and myofascial adhesions (section 4.2.3). As a result, the muscles involved become less elastic and movement becomes restricted. This leads to altered neuromuscular control. Your body looks for ways to compensate and changes its movement patterns, and other muscles are recruited to do the work of the injured muscle (this is known as synergistic dominance, section 3.6).

For example, you may begin to alter your running stride to compensate for an injured leg muscle that is tight and painful. Basically you are not using the correct muscles to control your movements. Unless the root cause of the problem is addressed, your soft tissue will adapt and begin to form permanent structural changes, causing muscle imbalances in that leg, which are going to result in the vicious circle. You will continue to alter your natural stride, and you will continue to be in pain and discomfort.

Muscle imbalance → Cumulative injury cycle → Tissue trauma → Inflammation → Muscle spasm → Muscle adhesions → Altered neuromuscular control → (Muscle imbalance)

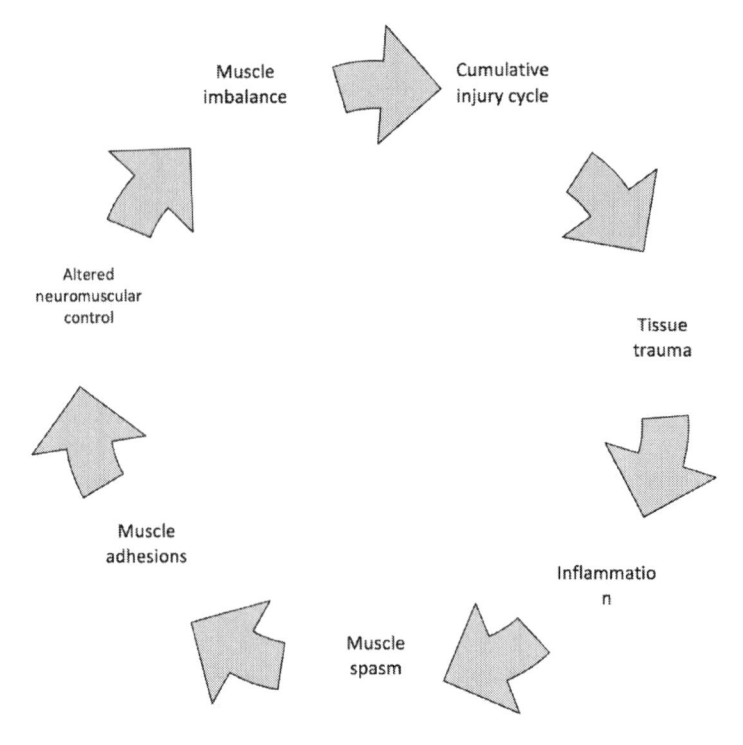

Diagram 6.2.8: The Cumulative Injury Cycle

Sample Corrective Exercises for Postural Dysfunctions

6.3 Corrective Exercises for Hyperlordosis

Hyperlordosis exists because of a muscular imbalance causing lower crossed syndrome (diagram 6.2.1). To correct hyperlordosis, the hip flexors need to be stretched along with the muscles of the lower back. The glutes and abdominals also need to be strengthened.

The following exercise guidelines are for information purposes only, and you should seek professional advice prior to embarking on these activities. Most of these exercises have been discussed in previous chapters, to which you will be referred accordingly.

Your exercise professional will specify the number of sets and repetitions depending upon your experience and personal needs. It must be emphasized that the core must be activated whilst performing these activities (section 4.4.2.3).

Hip Flexor Stretch

Please refer to section 4.3.2.2 for details on this stretch.

Lower Back Stretch

Apart from those stretches described in section 4.3.2.7, you can also try this back stretch (see diagram 6.3a below):

- Lie on your back with your knees bent.
- Pull your knees in towards your back as far as is comfortable.
- Hold the stretch for twenty to thirty seconds and repeat.

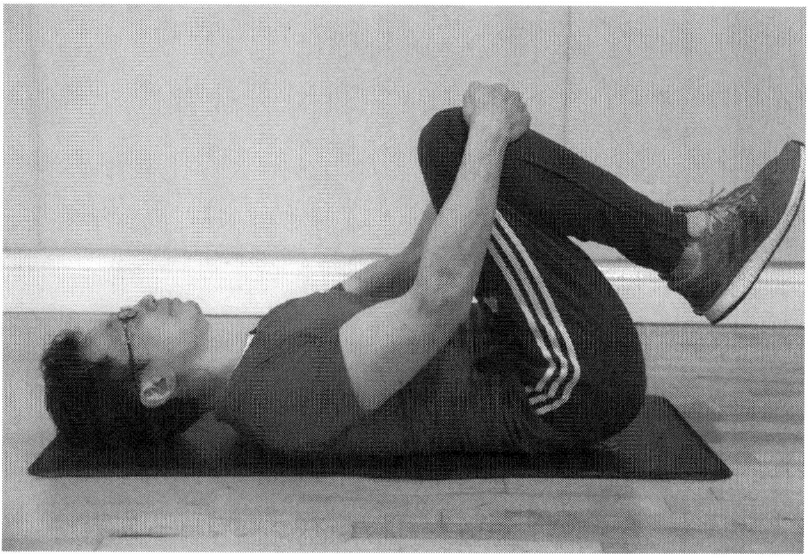

Diagram 6.3a: Lower Back Stretch

Apart from activating your transversus abdominis (section 4.4.2.3) and strengthening your core (section 4.4.3), you need to strengthen the other abdominal muscles ("abs"), such as your rectus abdominis:

Abdominal Crunch (Easy)

- Lie on your back with your knees bent at ninety degrees.
- Gently slide your hands up towards your knees and back down again, raising your head and shoulders off the floor but keeping your lower back firmly in position on the floor. You should be able to feel your abdominal muscles contracting.
- Repeat this exercise until you feel the stomach muscles working hard.
- Hold momentarily at the top and lower your shoulders slowly back to the ground. Repeat for the recommended number of repetitions advised by your trainer.

Abdominal Crunch (Harder, diagram 6.3b))

- You can increase the difficulty of this exercise by placing your hands across your chest or beside your head as shown below (but not behind your head, as this might strain your neck).
- You can challenge your core stability by performing the crunch on a Swiss ball (see diagram 6.3c). But ensure that your lower back stays in contact with the ball at all times.

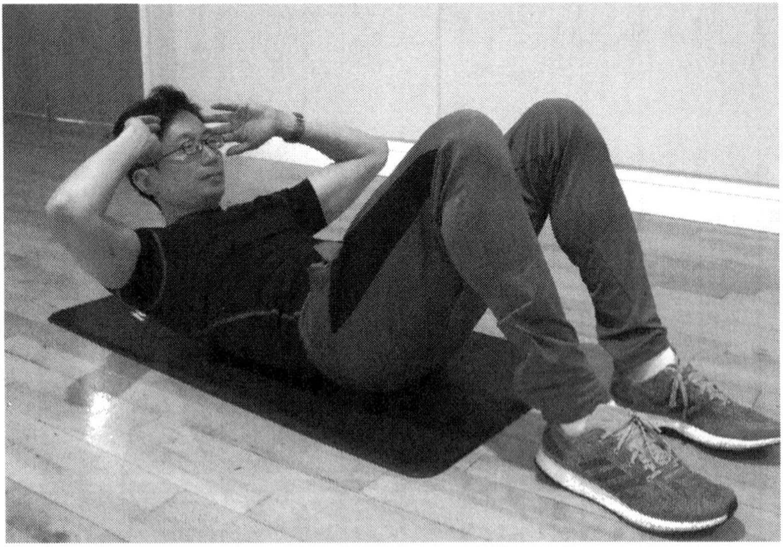

Diagram 6.3b: Abdominal Crunch

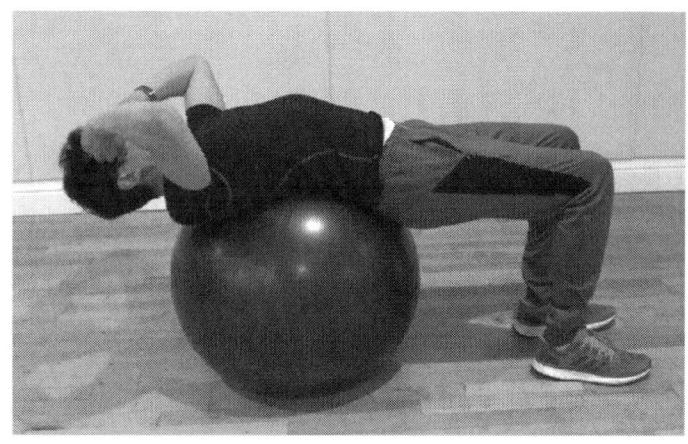

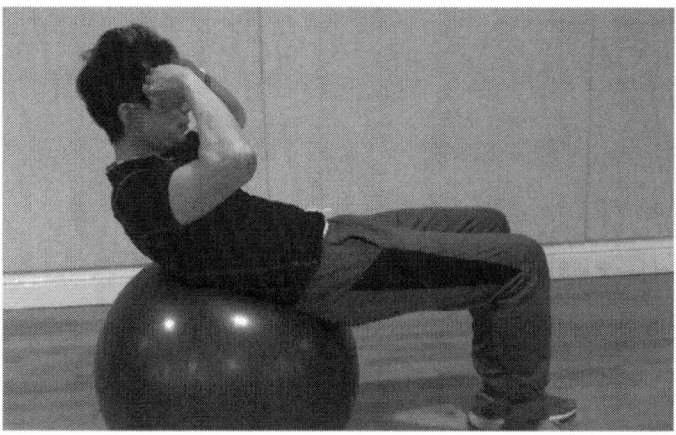

Diagram 6.3c: Abdominal Crunch on Stability Ball

Twisting Crunch

- Lie on your back with your knees bent and your feet flat on the floor.
- Position your hands by your temples.
- As you raise your head and shoulders up, ensure that your lower back is not raised but in constant contact with the floor. Twist your upper body so that your right elbow moves towards your left knee. Remember that this is not a sit-up.
- Return to the starting position and repeat, alternating between left and right twists.

Glute Bridge

Please refer to section 4.4.2.1 for details on this activation exercise.

6.4 Corrective Exercises for Hyperkyphosis

With postural hyperkyphosis/upper crossed syndrome, the tight pectorals, upper back and neck extensor muscles need to be stretched. Conversely, the weakened muscles, such as the middle trapezius, rhomboids and deep neck flexors, need to be strengthened.

Long periods of prolonged static posture with the head leaning forward and the shoulders protracted are prime contributory factors in such problems. Maintaining a good posture whilst working, combined with stretching and regular exercises, can greatly reduce the propensity for posture-related dysfunctions, such as neck and lower back pain.

Sample Strengthening Exercises for the Middle Trapezius and Rhomboids
---

- **Seated row (diagram 6.4a)**

    It is preferable to access the low pulley row machine with a V-bar; this enables you to have a neutral grip with the palms of your hands facing each other.

    - Sit down on the machine and place your feet on the front platform, slightly bending but not locking your knees.
    - Lean over and grab the V-bar handles.
    - To start with your arms extended, pull back the V-bar until your torso is at a ninety-degree angle from your legs. Your back should be slightly extended (arched backward), and your chest should be slightly protruding.
    - Engage your core, and by only flexing your elbows, pull the handles back towards the lower aspect of your sternum while keeping your torso stationary. At the top of the movement, maintain retraction of your shoulders and keep your upper

back hollow. Hold that contraction momentarily before slowly returning the V-bar to the original position.
- Repeat for the recommended number of repetitions advised by your trainer.

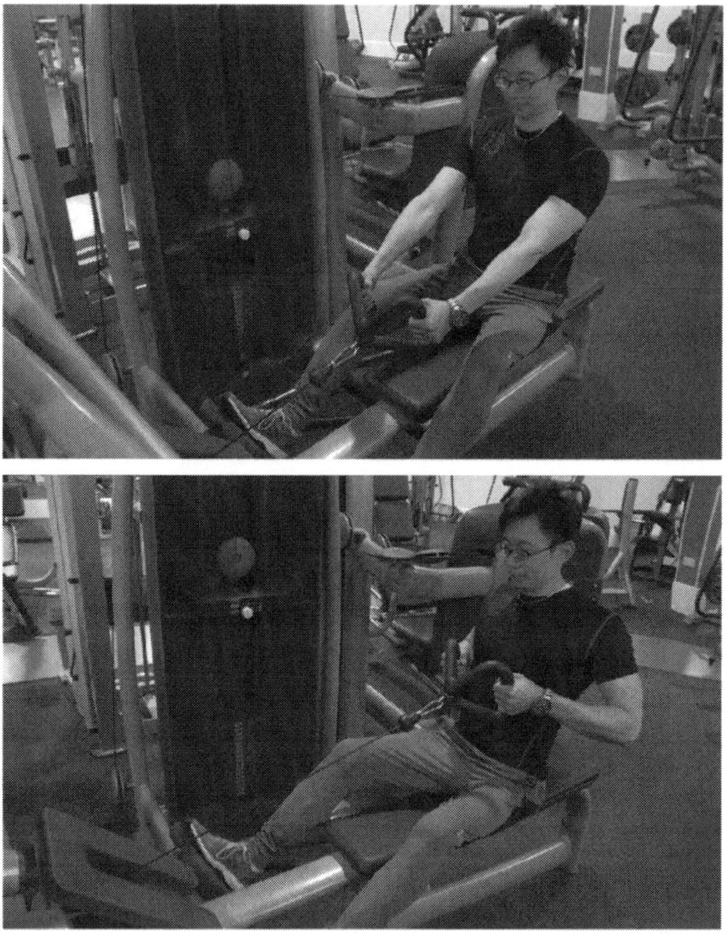

Diagram 6.4a – seated row

- **Single-Arm Dumb-bell Rows (diagram 6.4b)**

    - Start by standing next to a flat bench and position your left knee on the bench with a dumb-bell in your right hand.

- Pivot forward from your hips and place your left hand on the bench.
- Ensure that your upper body is straight and parallel to the floor with your head facing down.
- Your right hand, holding the dumb-bell, should hang straight down with the palm facing the bench.
- Keeping your arm close to the side of your body, engage your core and pull the dumb-bell up to your side. Take care not to twist your torso up whilst you lift the weight.
- Pause momentarily and then slowly lower the weight back to the starting position.
- Repeat for the recommended number of repetitions advised by your trainer until the set is finished.
- Switch arms and repeat.

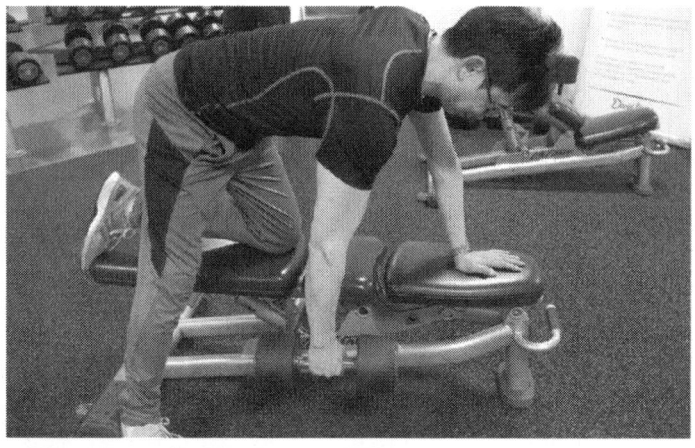

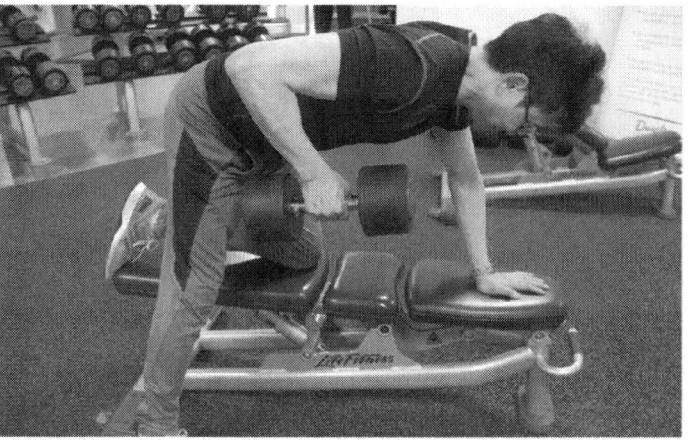

Diagram 6.4b: Single Arm Dumb-bell Row

- **Bent-Over Row (diagram 6.4c)**

  - Stand with your legs hip-width apart, with your knees slightly bent and your hips flexed forward (bend forward pivoting from your hips rather than by bending your lower back).
  - Hold the barbell with straight arms at around knee level, with your hands just wider than your knees on the bar and your palms facing down.
  - Keep your back stationary and engage your core as you pull the bar in towards your chest. Hold momentarily before slowly returning the bar to the starting position.

- Repeat for the recommended number of repetitions advised by your trainer.

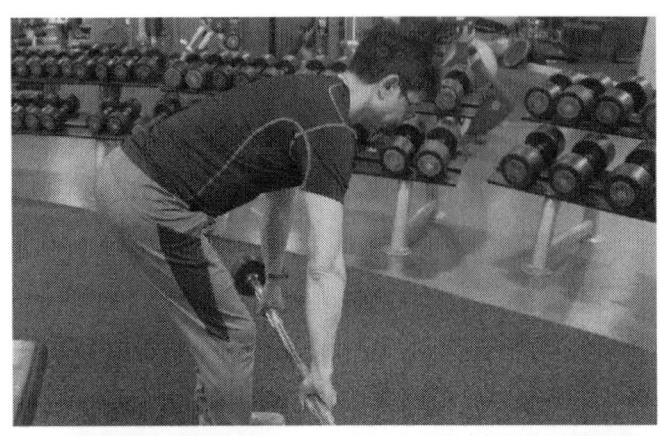

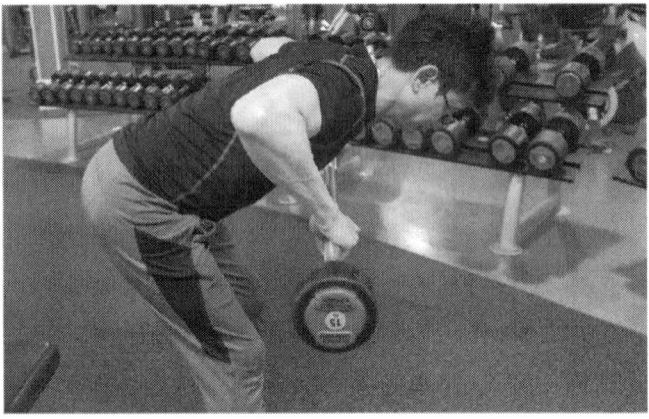

Diagram 6.4c bent over row

- **Reverse Fly (diagram 6.4d)**

  - To begin, lie down on an inclined bench with your chest and stomach pressing against it. Have a dumb-bell in each hand with your palms facing each other (neutral grip).
  - Keeping your arms slightly bent, lift the dumb-bells out to the sides of your body.

- At the top of the movement, maintain retraction of your shoulders and keep your upper back hollow before slowly lowering the dumbbells back down to the starting position.
- This completes one repetition. Repeat for the recommended number of repetitions advised by your trainer.

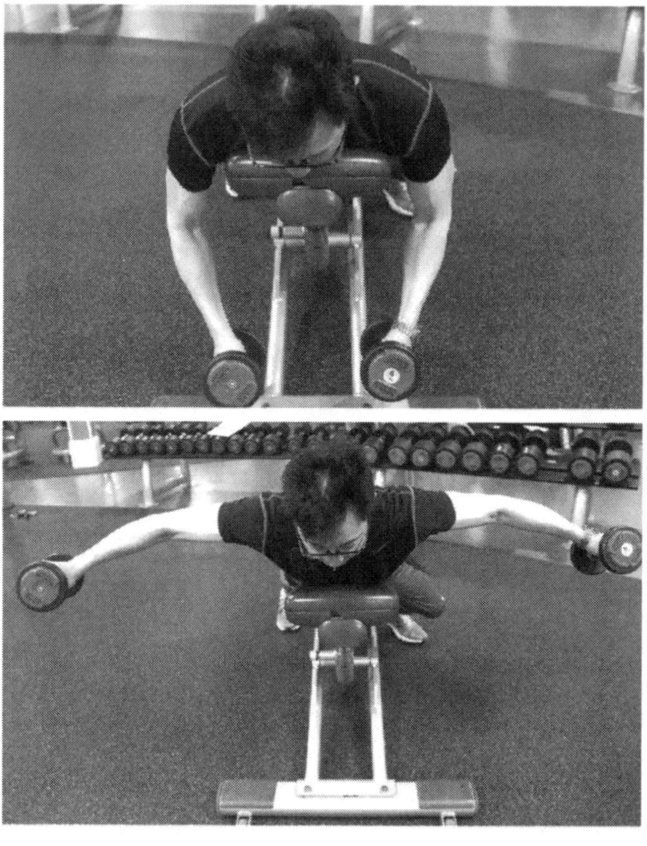

Diagram 6.4d: Reverse Fly

Pectoral Stretch (diagram 6.4e)

- Stand in a doorway or next to a wall.
- Bend the arm on the side to be stretched and place the forearm flat against a wall or doorframe.
- Step forward and rotate your body away from your outstretched arm.
- Hold for between ten and thirty seconds.

James Tang

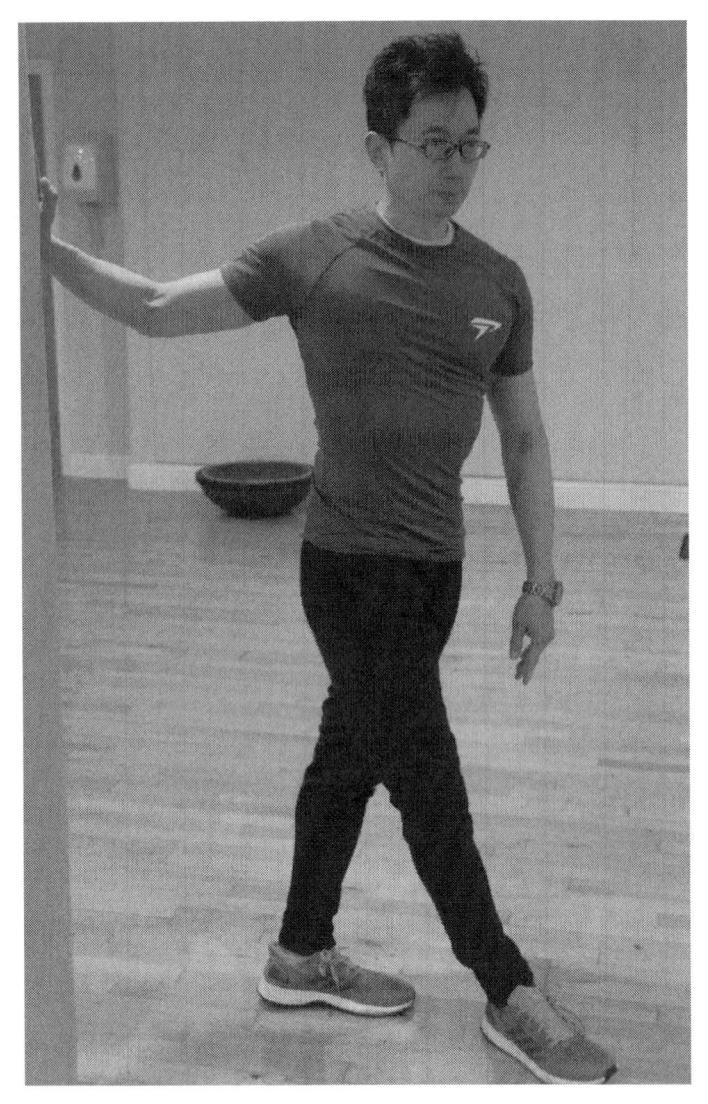

Diagram 6.4e: Pectoral Stretch

<u>Strengthening Exercise for the Deep Neck Flexors</u>

Weaknesses of the deep neck flexors are commonly associated with neck pain (similar to weaknesses of the transversus abdominis being commonly associated with lower back pain). Neck flexors can be activated by simple head-nodding motions (chin tucks), i.e., by moving the chin closer to your Adam's apple. This can improve both the strength and endurance of these deep muscles, which can in turn improve your posture and the biomechanics of your neck, shoulders, and upper limbs.

To perform chin tucks, stand against a wall so that when you retract your head, it just touches the wall. Hold this position while breathing normally for ten seconds, and repeat the process twelve to fifteen times. Hold the position longer as you become stronger. You should also feel some stretching in the muscles at the back of your neck at the same time.

Conclusion

You can do all the foam rolling, all the stretching and all the heavy weight training you want, but if your focus is not on improving your posture, nothing is likely to change. This is because your central nervous system gathers and interprets peripheral proprioceptive sensory information in order to execute the appropriate motor response. An individual with poor posture or who trains with an improper form will reinforce these bad habits by delivering improper sensory information to the central nervous system, which can lead to movement compensation. This is because the body will continually adapt in an attempt to produce the functional outcome that is requested by the system. Unfortunately, this adaptability will lead to muscle imbalance, dysfunction, and injury, such as lower back pain.

As previously mentioned, only a limited variety of corrective exercises have been mentioned and there are numerous alternatives available. It is clearly beyond the scope of this book to describe the detailed execution of these activities, such as the number of sets and repetitions. It is imperative that you engage an appropriate professional who can give you advice and guidance to ensure that the correct activities are being chosen for your particular situation.

Furthermore, you should not carry out any of the above corrective exercises until you have been properly assessed by your relevant professionals. Following a full postural assessment, a bespoke rectification programme will be designed for you, and guidance will be provided with regard to the execution of the corrective exercises.

It must be repeated that the author is not attempting to offer any diagnosis or treatment; he is providing general information purely from the perspective of an exercise professional, and this should not be considered as medical opinion.

CHAPTER 7

Flat Feet and Lower Back Pain

Introduction

You may be wondering why you are still suffering from recurrent back pain even though you take particular care of your posture and follow all the advice of your exercise professional, performing the correct stretches and exercises. If your trigger points recur in spite of adequate treatment, you need to look for the perpetuating factors, such as mechanical stressors that maintain them. For example, one of the perpetuators of your lower back predicament could be originating from as far down the kinetic chain as your feet.

Please be reminded that the human movement system (HMS) (section 2.8) is an integrated and multidimensional system. Impairment in one system can lead to compensation and adaptation in other systems, initiating the cumulative injury cycle (section 6.2.8) and resulting in decreased performance and injury, such as lower back pain.

During functional movements, the body must maintain its centre of gravity aligned over a constantly changing base of support. If a change in alignment occurs at one joint, changes in alignment at another joint must occur to compensate. You will be able to see from this chapter that the joint biomechanics of the ankle can affect the length-tension relationship (section 2.6) of the muscles that are attached to the lumbo-pelvic-hip complex, contributing to lower back pain. The reverse is also true; muscle imbalances of the hip can affect the lower extremities, contributing to knee pain and flat feet.

What Is Pronation?

Pronation is natural in the body's regular movement and occurs when weight is transferred from the heel to the toes during walking and running. The foot naturally rolls inward, and the medial arch flattens to provide shock absorption at the foot. The term "flat feet" is used to describe the effect of overpronation. The opposite movement to pronation is supination.

Overpronation can cause problems throughout your body because the overpronated foot is not properly absorbing the shock of your stride but instead transmitting that shock up through your knees and hips, which can have a profound effect on the balance and length-tension relationship of your lower back and pelvic musculatures.

Overpronating also forces the inner toes to take on all the work of pushing off for your next step. This can lead to other foot problems, such as plantar fasciitis (inflammation of the plantar fascia—the ligament that connects your heel bone to your toes and supports the arches of your foot).

As mentioned, it is natural for the foot to pronate during walking or running, and the tibia, knees, and hip correspondingly rotate internally. For individuals with overpronated feet, this internal rotation of the knees and hips is exaggerated (see diagram 8.1 below).

Furthermore, hyperpronation of the foot induces a compensatory anterior pelvic tilt, and this is correlated with hyperlordosis (section 6.2.1), which alters the length-tension relationship of the muscles that are attached to the lumbo-pelvic-hip complex. Over time, if this is not addressed, these imbalances can have a cumulative effect, causing a downward spiral which may eventually result in lower back pain (section 6.2.8).

Anterior pelvic tilt

Internal rotation of the hip

Internal rotation of the knees (knee valgus)

Hyperpronation of the foot

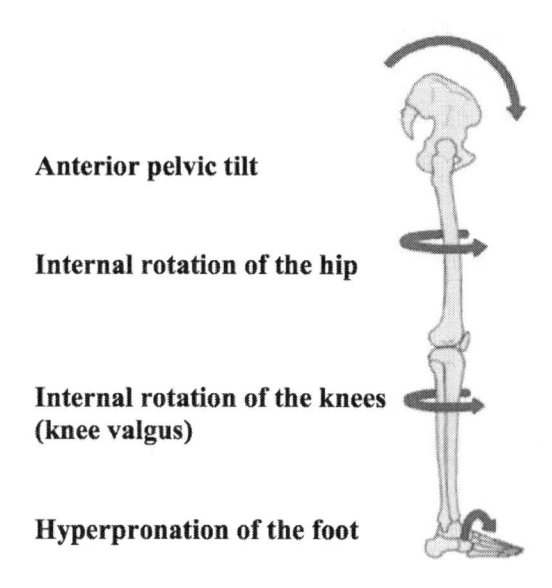

Diagram 8.1: Flat Foot with Internal Rotation of Knees and Anterior Pelvic Tilt

How Can I Tell If I Overpronate?

Firstly, conduct a static postural assessment. Take a look at your feet when you are standing and see whether you have a clear medial arch. If the inner sole touches the floor, then your feet are overpronated. Secondly, take a look at your running shoes. If they are worn down on the inside of the soles in particular, then you may have overpronation, or flat feet.

Normal Foot Arches

1. The medial longitudinal arch is the primary arch.
2. The lateral longitudinal arch runs along the outside of the foot and is not as deep or as wide or as long as the medial longitudinal arch.
3. The transverse arch runs across the bottom of the foot just proximal to the metatarsal heads. It traverses the ball of the foot at the front of the foot between the toes and the mid-foot.

Each of these arches, along with the bones, joints, ligaments, tendons and muscles, is designed to provide adequate support and flexibility for the foot.

Causes of Overpronation of the Foot

Walking on a Flat, Rigid and Unyielding Surface

Your feet were created to function on unpacked earth that yields with pressure and encourages normal dynamics of the bones, joints, ligaments, muscles, and arches because the earth is a natural arch support and shock absorber.

Your feet are not designed for standing or walking on hard, flat, and unyielding surfaces, such as concrete, wood, or carpeted floors. Your heel strikes the hard and unyielding surface (no shock absorption), causing forces to be transmitted up your body, through the knees, and up to the lumbo-pelvic-hip complex.

As you go into mid-stance where the entire foot is flat on the surface, there is no upward support for the three arches, causing them to collapse further than normal in order to meet the flat surface below. Finally, when you toe off, again there is no give in the surface, and forces are exerted into the toes and balls of the feet.

The body is efficient at adapting to stresses that are placed on it but it is not very smart. These adaptations, over time, cause muscle imbalance—the muscles around the ankle joint may become overactive in an attempt to minimize the stress at the involved segment.

Muscle Imbalances

Muscle imbalances are theorized to contribute to foot pronation[14], specifically tightness of the lateral ankle musculature including the lateral gastrocnemius, soleus, and peroneals. If the antagonistic muscles including the medial gastrocnemius, anterior tibialis, and posterior tibialis are weak, they may be unable to overcome the valgus joint positioning. You may therefore need to consult a corrective exercise specialist to identify the overactive muscles so that these can be deactivated with myofascial release and stretches. Similarly, underactive muscles can be activated through the prescription of a series of corrective exercises. For example, if there is weakness in the tibialis posterior, the most central and deepest of the calf muscles which help to support the medial arch of the foot, this muscle may need to be strengthened.

Summary

If you suffer from repeated episodes of back pain with no means of relief, apart from just paying attention to your back and glute musculatures, you may need to have your ankle alignment assessed as well. If you have flat feet, this may have contributed to the recurrence of your lower back pain. You need to seek advice from a podiatrist who can prescribe you with orthotic devices that can correct your lower extremity movement impairment syndrome.

Foot orthotics can help manage lower back pain by improving and stabilizing the position of the feet, which in turn improves every aspect of the HMS kinetic chain. The feet represent the base of the kinetic chain, and each subsequent joint above the feet can be considered to be a link in this chain, which goes all the way up the trunk of the body to the neck.

Again, the purpose of this chapter is to merely highlight to you that what happens down in your feet can affect the structures all the way up to your hips, lower back, and even your neck and shoulders. You are reminded that you should seek help from an appropriate professional in order to identify the root cause of your musculoskeletal lower back disorder.

CHAPTER 8

Sacroiliac Joint Dysfunction and Lower Back Pain

8.1 Functional Anatomy of the Sacroiliac Joints (SI joints)

The sacroiliac (SI) joints are located at the sacrum (*a triangle-shaped bone made up of five vertebrae fused together near the bottom of your spine, just above your coccyx, or tailbone*) and they join the spine to the ilium (*one of the three bones that make up your pelvis/hip bones, is the uppermost point of your pelvis*) on either side through small, strong ligaments. In addition, there are a number of strong muscles that surround the SI joints, including the erector spinae, psoas, quadratus lumborum, piriformis, abdominal obliques, gluteals, and the hamstrings. However, none of these muscles actually act directly on the SI joints to produce active movements. Instead, movements are produced indirectly by gravity and by these muscles acting on the trunk and lower limbs.

The bones of the SI joints are jagged, which helps them to stay in alignment. The SI joints are synovial anteriorly (meaning it is filled with synovial fluid, which provides lubrication) and fibrous posteriorly, allowing only minimal movement in flexion and extension of your pelvis and lower spine.

The SI joints primarily move in the saggital plane (front and back), and this is necessary for normal functional activities. Their main role is to support the weight of your upper body when you stand or walk and to transmit that load to your legs. They act as a shock absorber and reduce the pressure on your spine. They must also support your body when you twist or when you lift objects. Because your SI joints transfer compressive forces during weight-bearing activities, they must remain stable. Muscles that are attached to the lumbo-pelvic-hip complex, as well as the core musculatures (the diaphragm, transverse abdominis, multifidus, and pelvic floor muscles [section 3.3.2.2]), help to support the SI joints and provide pelvic stability.

8.2 Causes of SI Joint Pain

Muscle imbalances affect the SI joints, even though none of these muscles directly act on the joints. When the muscles that are attached to the lumbo-pelvic-hip complex, both above and below the SI joints, are balanced and working in synchrony, we maintain a neutral posture that is "stress-free", as the muscles supporting the spine and hips are at their correct length-tension relationships (section 2.6), meaning that they are able to produce the right amount of force at the right time and in the right direction.

When the muscles around the SI joints become imbalanced (section 3.2), commonly through poor postural habits (section 6.2), overuse, or poor body mechanics, such as prolonged sitting or a poor sitting posture (e.g. sitting with crossed legs or prolonged sitting with a wallet in the back pocket on one side), the muscles surrounding the them become overused, overactive, or overly tight, and others become underused, underactive, and overly lengthened. When this happens, unequal stress is being placed on the hips and spine. For instance, tension in the piriformis through the formation of trigger points (section 4.3.2.5) can put a twist in the SI joints. Trigger points are particularly prevalent in the piriformis either through overuse, as in strenuous training, or underuse, as in excessive sitting. Tight hamstrings can also cause the hips and pelvis to rotate back, flattening the lower back and causing back problems and SI joint pain.

The body senses this stress as an injury and begins the inflammation process in an attempt to heal the joint, thereby producing swelling and pain. Inflammation of one or both SI joints is called sacroiliac joint dysfunction. If the stimulus for injury and inflammation is not attended to, pain and swelling will continue, joint tissue will subsequently wear down (causing osteoarthritis), and chronic pain will persist.

Gout can occur if your body has high levels of uric acid. This disease is characterized by joint pain. Although gout almost always affects the large toe first, all joints can be affected, including the SI joints.

Relaxin, a hormone released during pregnancy, makes the SI joints more flexible. This enables the pelvis to widen to accommodate the birth of a baby. However, it also renders the joints more unstable. Combined with weight gain and the weight of the baby, this often leads to SI joint pain. Women who experience this are more prone to getting arthritis in the SI joints—a risk that increases with each pregnancy.

Walking abnormally can cause SI joint dysfunction. You may walk abnormally because of issues such as uneven leg lengths or flat feet (chapter 7).

SI Joints can also be damaged due to **traumas**, such as injuries resulting from sports, falls or car accidents.

Ankylosing spondylitis is a type of inflammatory arthritis that affects the vertebrae and joints of the spine. In severe cases, ankylosing spondylitis can cause new bone growth that fuses the joints in the spine.

8.3 Symptoms and Diagnosis of SIJ Problems

SI joint pain varies but you may experience a sharp, stabbing pain that radiates from your hips and pelvis, up to the lower back, and down to the thighs. Sometimes it may feel numb or tingly. The lower back often feels stiff when getting up after sitting for long periods and when getting out of bed in the morning; you may even experience pain in your lower back when you stand up from your chair. You often feel the pain on one side of your lower back. Like other musculoskeletal lower back pain, pain tends to be more intense in the morning but often gets better during the day.

The SI joints are implicated in 15 to 30 per cent of cases of chronic lower back pain.

Diagnosing SI Joint Problems

SI joint problems are often difficult to diagnose because these joints are located deep in your body, making it difficult for your doctor to examine or test their motion. Often, damage to the joints does not show up on imaging tests, such as X-rays, MRIs, or CT scans, and the symptoms often resemble those of sciatica, bulging discs, and arthritis of the hip.

Your doctor may have to inject a numbing drug into the SI joint. If the pain then disappears, this indicates that you most likely have an SI joint problem.

8.4 Corrective Exercises for Lower Back Pain Resulting from SI Joint Dysfunction

As with any self-help corrective exercise protocol, you must seek professional advice prior to embarking on these exercises, and supervision by an exercise professional is of the utmost importance.

Although the SI joints are meant to be extremely stable joints, slight movement is crucial in order for them to absorb the large forces headed for your lumbar vertebrae. Stabilization of the SI joints comes from the muscles that surround them and problems can arise when there is either too much or too little movement in the joints, often resulting from imbalances in these muscles.

All muscles that are attached to the lumbo-pelvic-hip complex can influence the function of the SI joints to a varying extent. The objective of any corrective exercise is to reverse muscle imbalances so as to remove restriction and improve mobility of the SI joints. For instance, stretching the muscles serves to restore a normal range of motion, improve muscle imbalances around the SI joints and reduce tension in the overactive muscles which can pull the SI joints out of place.

The most effective way of treating SI pain is to engage in an corrective exercise programme specific to correcting poor postural habits (sections 6.3 and 6.4), increasing flexibility of the overly tight muscles (section 4.3), increasing the activity of the under-active muscles (section 4.4), and then learning how to maintain proper core stability (section 4.5.1) and joint alignment throughout all of your recreational or daily activities. This includes working the abdominals (sections 4.4.2.3 and 4.4.3) and the muscles surrounding the spine, hips, and shoulder blades. As part of this process, it is vital that you are aware of your daily postural habits (chapter 6).

Furthermore, rest after engaging in any activities that cause pain, such as running. You may be advised to wear a sacroiliac support belt, which may help take the strain off the joints and provide relief from symptoms.

Again, as this is not a medical textbook, the author can only recommend corrective exercises to alleviate your back problems. Medical options such as steroid injections, anti-inflammatory drugs and surgery are beyond the scope of this book. It is important to reiterate that if you suffer from any form of back pain, you must seek medical advice in order to establish a correct diagnosis.

Conclusion

Please be aware that there are other corrective exercises for SI joint dysfunction and that such activities are not designed to be a stand-alone programme but are instead a guide to help you understand the direction a therapeutic exercise approach to the SI joints should take. This may assist you, your exercise professional, doctor, physiotherapist, sports therapist, or chiropractor with some potential options for how to support the process of restoring your overall health and function.

CHAPTER 9

The Best Way to Sleep for Lower Back Pain Sufferers

9.1 Ideal Sleep Positions to Ease Your Lower Back Pain

If you suffer from musculoskeletal pain, the real culprit may not be your sleeping position but your daily activities, or the lack of them. You should take measures during the day to avoid prolonged sitting; try to vary your posture as much as possible and consciously maintain good posture when standing and sitting. These measures will go a long way to helping you to reduce your nocturnal musculoskeletal discomforts.

For most musculoskeletal pain sufferers, the discomfort can make it difficult to enjoy a good night's sleep. At the same time, how you sleep may exacerbate your condition. This is because while certain sleeping positions put a strain on already aching tissues, others may help you find relief. It must be remembered that we are all different; similar to corrective exercises, there is no one-size-fits-all sleeping position for pain sufferers. Like any other prolonged static postures, any sleeping position has the potential to amplify your pain if you maintain it for too long; it is therefore advantageous to move around and change your sleeping position where possible, because a little movement can help ease the pressure on your back and neck.

Sleeping on Your Back

This is the best position for keeping your back pain under control, because it offers optimal support to your spine and helps to maintain its natural curvatures (section 6.1) so that it can rest naturally, especially if you sleep without a pillow. Furthermore, sleeping on your back evenly distributes weight across the widest surface of your body, minimizing pressure points and ensuring proper alignment of your internal organs. Ensure your mattress is not too soft; a medium-firm or firm mattress can help provide support. Unfortunately, too many people sleep on a mattress that is far too soft for this purpose.

If you sleep with a pillow, ensure that it fills the space between your neck and the mattress so your head maintains a neutral position. However, if you sleep on too many pillows, this can cause your head to jut forward of your shoulders all night, similar to the detrimental forward head posture (section 6.2.2) that many of us maintain all day in front of our computers.

Many people, lie on their back with their knees fully extended (straight) and this can create lower back strain because this position pulls the pelvis out of its normal alignment. Sleeping all night in this hyperlordotic position (section 6.2.1) may tighten your lower back muscles, resulting in a predisposition to back pain. To overcome this problem, you can try supporting the back of your knees by putting a pillow under them; your legs are likely rest in a slightly bent position, which in turn will encourage a more neutral pelvic position.

Sleeping on Your Stomach (prone position)

Sleeping on your stomach is problematic for most people, especially those with lower back pain, because it creates stress on the back muscles by accentuating your lumbar lordotic curve (section 6.2.1), causing unnecessary tension in the muscles that are attached to the lumbo-pelvic-hip complex.

Furthermore, it is inevitable that your head will be rotated to one side or the other, predisposing you to neck pain. The best advice is to avoid stomach sleeping altogether, but if this is not possible, you may wish to consider putting a flat pillow under your abdomen to help lengthen your lower back curve by elevating the hips a little to relieve the strain across the back and relax the muscles. You can also consider not using a pillow for your head, in order to allow your head to rest in good alignment during the night.

Sleeping on Your Side

This position can lead to back and hip problems because the top leg slides forward, causing the lower portion of your spine to rotate. Also, some side sleepers' top shoulder droops forward while they sleep, creating a unilateral hyperkyphotic posture, and causing more spinal rotation.

Try to draw your legs up slightly towards your chest and sleep with a pillow between your knees; this will help keep your whole body aligned while you sleep. In addition, consider positioning your pillow so that part of it is under your neck, and therefore fills in the space between your neck and the bed, providing more support for your neck curve.

9.2 Pillow Strategies

Choosing **supportive cervical pillows** is beneficial since you spend about a third of your day sleeping. This time could be spent helping your neck posture if you utilize a proper pillow support for your neck. Pillows that are too soft and too large can cause problems. To support your neck, your head should rest on a small, hard pillow.

Whichever sleeping position you choose, position your pillow beneath your head and neck, and not your shoulders. You may prefer to use a contoured pillow to alleviate neck strain or to sleep on just one pillow instead of a stack of several pillows.

Pillows can support your head during sleep, which in turn will help you relax and therefore avoid muscle or joint strain to vulnerable areas. If you have lower back or neck pain, it is advisable to test different types of pillows as a way of reducing strain around the vertebral joints.

9.3 Mattresses for Lower Back Pain

To avoid neck and back pain, it is important to select a good mattress that supports your body. It should be elastic at every point, and it should not sink under the pelvis, shoulder, or head.

Sleeping on the wrong mattress can cause or worsen back pain. A Lack of support from a mattress reinforces a poor sleeping posture, strains muscles, and does not help to maintain the correct spinal alignment, all of which can contribute to lower back pain. A mattress that provides both comfort and back support helps to reduce back pain, allowing the structures of the spine to rest naturally during the night.

Following is some practical advice to help those with lower back pain to choose the best mattress for both back support and sleep comfort:

- It is really a matter of personal preference, because there is no single mattress style or type that works for everyone with back pain. Any mattress that helps you sleep without pain and stiffness is the best mattress for you. It is therefore advisable to try before you buy.

- Overall comfort is equally as important as sufficient back support. Sleeping on a mattress that is too firm can cause aches and pains on pressure points. A medium-firm mattress may be more comfortable because it allows the shoulders and hips to sink slightly. Ultimately, it is your body type that dictates the type of support you need. If your hips are wider than your waist, a softer mattress can accommodate the width of your pelvis and allow your spine to remain neutral. If your hips and waist are in a relatively straight line, a more rigid surface will offer better support.

- Know when it is time to get a new mattress. If an old mattress sags visibly in the middle or is no longer comfortable, it is probably time to purchase a new one. Placing a hard board under the mattress to keep it from sagging in the middle is not a viable long-term solution.

FURTHER READING

Active IQ, *Level 3 Personal Training Manual.*
Active IQ, *Level 3 Sports Massage Therapy Manual.*
Active IQ, *Level 4 Sports Massage Therapy Manual.*
Bean, Anita, The Complete Guide to Sports Nutrition, 4th edition.
Coulson, Morc, The Fitness Instructor's Handbook, 2nd edition.
—— and David Archer, *The Advanced Fitness Instructor's Handbook.*
Davies, Clair, *The Trigger Point Therapy Workbook*, 2nd ed.
Gibbons, John, *Muscle Energy Techniques—A Practical Guide for Physical Therapists.*
Lawrence, Debbie, The Complete Guide to Exercise Referral.
Lawrence, Matt, *The Complete Guide to Core Stability*, 3rd edition.
Niel-Asher, Simeon, *The Concise Book of Trigger Points—A Professional and Self-Help Manual*, 3rd ed.
Norris, Christopher M., The Complete Guide to Stretching, 3rd edition.
Paine, Tim, The Complete Guide to Sports Massage, 3rd edition.
Patel, Kesh, The Complete Guide to Postural Training.
Priso, Anada, *An Introductory Guide to Cupping Therapy.*
Starlanyl, Devub J., and John Sharkey, *Healing Through Trigger Point Therapy—A Guide to Fibromyalgia, Myofascial Pain and Dysfunction.*
Waddell, Gordon, *The Back Pain Revolutions.*
Ward, Keith, *Hands On Sports Therapy.*

INDEX

Abdominal bracing 101
Abdominal crunches 107, 114, 122
Abdominal crunch 187, 188, 189
Abdominal obesity 18, 40, 89, 116, 122, 177
Abductors 70, 82, 84
Accessory movements 22
Acetylcholine 10, 46
Acromion process 174
Actin 6, 10, 11, 46
Activation phase 41, 93
Active rest 126, 137, 138, 144
Active stretch 78
Active trigger points 52, 69, 70
Acupuncture 35, 46
Adaptation 75, 109, 141, 142, 143, 151, 155, 156, 158, 199, 202
Adductor longus 82
Adductors 25, 39, 77, 82
Adenosine diphosphate (ADP) 125
Adhesions 35, 42, 44, 45, 71, 72, 185
Adrenal cortex 128
Adrenaline 140
Aerobic 6, 7, 142, 145, 151, 156
Aerobic system 125, 126, 136, 140, 142
Age-related hyperkyphosis 178
Agonist 16, 28, 29, 30, 78, 154, 155, 159, 164

All-or-none law 9
Anabolism 118
Anaerobic 7, 125, 126, 130, 135, 136, 139, 141, 142, 151
Anaerobic glycolysis 139, 142, 151
Anaerobic threshold 135
Ankylosing spondylitis 206
Antagonist 16, 28, 29, 30, 41, 64, 76, 78, 80, 155, 164, 165, 176, 178, 202
Anterior inferior iliac spine (AIIS) 92
Anterior longitudinal ligaments 21
Anterior oblique subsystem 25
Anterior pelvic tilt xiii, xiv, 31, 40, 91, 101, 110, 116, 175, 177, 184, 200, 201
Anterior superior iliac spine (ASIS) 100, 173
Arthritis xviii, 38, 47, 74, 98, 115, 117, 169, 206, 207
Ascending pyramid 165, 166
ATP (Adenosine triphosphate) 8, 10, 11, 124, 125, 126, 138, 139, 140, 141, 142, 144
Attachment trigger points 46, 51
Autogenic inhibition 53
Axon 10

Back extension 114

Balance training 154
Ballistic stretch 78
Basal metabolic rate 118, 119, 122
Bent-over row 193
Bicep curl 27, 28, 29, 108, 114, 154, 157, 159, 164, 166
Bicep femoris 25, 78
Biceps 19, 27, 28, 29, 154, 155, 157, 158, 159
Biceps brachii 27, 28, 29, 159
Bicycle crunch 107
Biological value (BV) 123
Blood pooling 146
Blood pressure adaptation 156
Body composition 74, 117, 156
Body composition adaptation 156
Bone tissue adaptation 156
Bosu ball 112
Brachialis 29
Brachioradialis 29
Bradykinin 46
Brevis 82

Calcium 10, 11, 46
Calf 9, 46, 78
Calorie 100, 101118, 119, 121, 122, 124, 126, 127, 128, 129, 134, 137, 138, 139, 140, 141, 147
Carbohydrates 119, 120, 121, 123, 124, 125, 126, 127, 128, 129, 132, 138, 140, 147
Cardiac muscle 5, 6
Cardiovascular fitness 74, 108, 137, 142, 145, 152
Catabolism 118, 167
Cervical lordosis 172
Chin tuck 196, 197
Chronic back pain xviii, 3, 47
Coccyx 66, 172, 204
Cold treatment 34

Compound exercises 141, 157
Concentric 62, 156, 159, 160, 162, 163, 164
Congenital hyperkyphosis 178
Cool-down 146
Core dysfunction 16, 19, 26, 27, 64, 100
Core muscles 7, 19, 26, 27, 62, 100, 108, 110, 111, 148
Core musculatures 7, 19, 27, 100, 107, 108, 110, 205
Core stability xii, 20, 21, 23, 27, 89, 95, 105, 106, 108, 109, 110, 111, 112, 114, 115, 153, 169, 170, 188, 208, 213
Corrective exercise continuum 41, 47
Corticosteroid 128
Cortisol 128
Creatine 124, 125, 140, 144
Cross-bridge 10, 11
Cumulative injury cycle 13, 26, 45, 184, 185, 186, 199
Cupping therapy 71, 213

Dead lifts 96
Deep longitudinal subsystem 25
Deep neck flexors 179, 181, 190, 196
Deep stroking massage 57, 73
Deltoids 19, 29, 155, 157, 162, 163
Depolarization 10
Descending pyramid 166
Developmental stretch 80
Diaphragm 7, 22, 24, 100, 109, 205
Diffuse trigger points 51
Dowager's hump 178
Drop set 163, 165
Dry needling 73
Dynamic stretch 55, 77, 78, 113, 148, 149
Dynamic stretches 77, 148

Eatwell plate 119, 120
Eccentric 30, 62, 70, 153, 156, 159, 160, 162, 163, 164
Ectomorph 151, 167, 168
Emotional stresses 15
Endomorph 168, 169
Endomysium 43
Epimysium 43
Erector spinae 25, 30, 31, 39, 49, 59, 60, 61, 62, 64, 78, 89, 90, 91, 176, 180, 204,
Excess post-exercise oxygen consumption (EPOC) 130
External obliques 24, 64

Fartlek 137, 143
Fascia 23, 25, 42, 200
Fascicle 43
Fast glycolytic fibres 8
Fast-twitch (Type 2) fibres 7
Fat 7, 111, 118, 119, 121, 122, 123, 124, 125, 126, 127, 128, 129, 130, 132, 134, 135, 137, 138, 139, 140, 142, 147, 156, 161, 162, 167, 168, 169
Fat-burning zone 138
Femoral trochlea 48
Femur 51, 66, 67, 70, 80, 92
Fibromyalgia 55, 213
Fixator 29, 108, 154
Flat back posture 79, 184
Flat feet xiv, 40, 54, 173, 199, 200, 201, 203, 206
Flexibility xii, 1, 16, 18, 20, 33, 34, 39, 43, 44, 74, 75, 76, 77, 82, 93, 108, 145, 152, 202, 208, 215
Flexibility tests 39
Flexor 8, 17, 29, 31, 39, 64, 65, 75, 77, 80, 81, 84, 86, 91, 92, 94, 111, 176, 179, 181, 186, 190, 196Foam roller 44, 53, 55, 60, 61, 66, 70
Forced reps 163
Forward head posture 19, 178. 180, 181, 184, 210
Free weights 153, 154, 170
Full pyramid 166

Gastrocnemius 202
Giant set – the Big G 161
Glenoid fossa 6
Global muscular system 7, 21
Glucose metabolism adaptation 156
Glute bridge 94, 95, 96, 190
Gluteal xviii, 20, 64, 65, 66, 68, 70, 86, 94, 204
Gluteal tuberosity 66
Glutes xiv, 8, 30, 39, 49, 64, 65, 75, 80, 81, 86, 90, 91, 94, 96, 97, 105, 141, 157, 176, 177, 186
Gluteus maximus 9, 17, 25, 39, 66, 67, 70, 71, 78, 84, 93, 94, 176
Gluteus medius 25, 39, 51, 64, 67, 68, 69, 84, 94, 98
Glycaemic index 121, 147
Glycogen 120, 121, 123, 125, 126, 127, 128, 135, 139, 140, 141, 144
Golgi tendon organs (GTO) 53
Gout 206
Gracilis 82
Greater sciatic foramen 70
Greater trochanter 51, 67, 70, 71, 174
Groin 63, 82
Ground substance 44

Haemoglobin 132, 140
Hamstring 67, 75, 77, 78, 79, 80, 94, 155, 157, 204, 205

Hamstrings 9, 16, 20, 25, 30, 39, 66, 75, 77, 78, 79, 80, 90, 91, 94, 157, 204, 205
Heart rate adaptation 156
Heat treatment 33
Herat rate reserve 133
Herniated discs 172
Hip flexors 8, 17, 30, 39, 65, 75, 77, 80, 81, 84, 86, 94, 111, 176, 186
Homeostasis 139
Human Movement System (HMS) 13, 26, 185, 199
Humerus 6
Hyperkyphosis 19, 40, 93, 155, 178, 179, 180, 182, 184, 190
Hyperlordosis xiii, xiv, 17
Hypertension 96, 156
Hypertrophy 115, 149, 150, 151, 152, 155, 156, 160, 161
Hypoglycaemia 121

Iliac crest 62, 66, 67, 69, 98, 100, 173
Iliacus 80
Iliocostalis 60, 61
Iliopsoas 30, 64, 80, 91, 176, 177
Iliotibial band (ITB) 66, 84, 98
Ilium 60, 204
Infrared lights 33
Infraspinatus 19
Inguinal ligament 100
Inhibitory phase 41, 42, 74
Inner range-holding tests 39
Insulin 121, 127, 129, 140, 142, 147, 156
Integration phase 41
Internal obliques 7, 64
Interspinales 22
Interspinous ligaments 21

Intertransversarii 22
Intertransverse ligaments 21
Interval training 126, 130, 137, 138, 141, 142, 143, 145, 161
Intervertebral discs xviii, 15, 33, 181
Intra-abdominal pressure 22, 23, 110
Intramuscular glycogen 121, 125, 126, 128, 139, 140
Ischemic compression 57
Ischial tuberosity 78
Isolated exercise 157
Isometric 100, 101, 102, 107, 108, 160, 162
Isotonic contraction 159
ITB syndrome 84
Iyengar Yoga 93

Karvonen method 133

Lactate system 125, 139
Lactic acid 125, 126, 135, 139, 140, 141, 142, 144, 146
Latent trigger points 52, 61, 66, 171
Lateral longitudinal arch 201
Lateral malleolus 174
Lateral pelvic tilt 31
Lateral stabilization 67
Lateral subsystem 25
Latissimus dorsi 24, 25, 157, 178
Lengthening phase 41, 74
Length-tension relationship 11, 12, 179
Levator scapulae 179, 181
Linea alba 100
Local muscular system 6, 22
Longissimus 60
Lower crossed syndrome 176, 177, 186
Lumbar lordosis 172, 184

Lumbo-pelvic-hip complex 12, 17, 18, 31, 33, 62, 80, 108, 175, 199, 200, 202, 205, 207, 210
Lunges 25, 96

Macronutrients 116, 118, 119, 120, 124, 126
Magnus 82
Maintenance stretch 79, 80
Matrix 21 166
Mattress 64, 210, 212
Maximum heart rate (MHR) 126, 132, 133, 138, 144
Medial longitudinal arch 201
Meridians 46
Mesomorph 151, 168
Microwavable heat belts 33
Military posture 184
Mitochondria 6, 7, 8
Motor end plate 10
Motor nerve 10
Motor unit 9, 10, 155
Movement assessments 38
Multipennate muscles 51
Muscle adaptation 12
Muscle dysfunction 2, 12, 17, 26, 180
Muscle failure 163
Muscle fibre adaptation 156
Muscle imbalance 16, 39, 40, 41, 42, 45, 75, 76, 99, 108, 116, 171, 174, 175, 177, 179, 185, 197, 202, 205, 207, 208
Muscle strength 75, 108
Muscle synergies 24, 25
Muscular endurance 74, 149, 151, 152, 153
Muscular strength 74, 112, 159
Musculoskeletal back pain 4, 38, 47
Musculoskeletal lower back pain 3, 4, 14, 16, 19, 63, 207

Myofascia 13, 41, 42, 43, 44, 50, 52, 54, 55, 56, 61, 71, 74, 182, 185, 203
Myofascial pain syndrome 42, 55
Myofibril 6, 10, 44, 45, 49
Myofilaments 10, 46
Myoglobin 6, 7, 8, 140
Myosin 6, 10, 11, 46

NASM – National Academy of Sports Medicine 41
Negative sets 163, 164
Neurological hyperkyphosis 178
Neuromuscular efficiency 13, 94, 115
Neuromuscular junction 10
Neuron 9
Neurotransmitter 10, 46
Neutral spine 19, 65, 94, 172
Neutralizer 29, 112
Nicotine 16
Nociceptors 46, 177
Noradrenaline 140

Obesity 18, 40, 89, 110, 116, 117, 122, 137, 147, 177
One-repetition maximum, 1 rep max (1RM) 151, 163
Onset of blood lactate accumulation (OBLA) 126, 141
Osteoarthritis 13, 47, 48, 50, 52, 117, 206
Osteoporosis 4, 75, 117
Overpronation 200, 201, 202
Oxygen debt 139, 140, 141, 142

Painkillers xi, 35
Passive stretch 78
Patella 48, 80, 84, 92, 98
Pectineus 82
Pectoral stretch 195, 196

Pectorals 19, 40, 155, 157, 160, 178, 179, 190
Pelvic floor muscles 7, 24, 100, 109, 110, 205
Perimysium 43
Peroneals 202
Phosphocreatine 124, 125, 140
Physiological movements 22
Physiotherapy 35
Pilates 93
Pillow 210, 211
Piriformis 30, 39, 49, 69, 70, 71, 77, 86, 87, 204, 205
Piriformis syndrome 70, 86, 87
Plank 99, 100, 101, 102, 103, 104, 105, 106, 107, 109, 160
Plantar fascia 200
Plantar fasciitis 200
Podiatrist xiv, 40, 203
Posterior deltoid 25
Posterior longitudinal ligaments 21
Posterior oblique subsystem 25
Posterior pelvic tilt 31, 79, 101, 173, 175, 179, 184
Posterior superior iliac spine (PSIS) 173
Post-exhaustion 162
Postural assessment 38, 173, 197, 201
Postural dysfunction xii, xiv, 17, 19, 40, 50, 54, 76, 171, 178, 186
Postural muscles 7, 9, 17, 19, 39, 54, 57, 77, 112, 176
Power stroke 11
Pre-exhaustion 162
Primary trigger points 51, 54
Prime mover 27, 28, 29, 30, 76, 86, 108, 114
Progression xiv, 48, 77, 95, 101, 103, 105, 109, 115, 152, 158, 182

Prolonged sitting 18, 26, 30, 31, 43, 50, 63, 64, 66, 68, 75, 76, 80, 84, 86, 98, 100, 137, 176, 177, 205, 209
Pronation 200, 202
Proprioceptive neuromuscular facilitation (PNF) 78
Protein 6, 11, 119, 121, 123, 124, 126, 127, 128, 129, 138, 144
Protein supplements 123
Psoas major 77, 80, 81, 111
Pubic crest 100
Pyramid set 165, 166

Quadratus lumborum 25, 30, 62, 69, 78, 88, 93, 99, 176, 204
Quadriceps 9, 16, 48, 65, 80, 91, 155, 157, 162

Rang-of-motion tests 38
Reciprocal inhibition 29, 30, 41, 64, 81, 84, 86, 94, 176, 181
Rectus abdominis – 20, 180, 187, 20, 23, 24, 26, 27, 31, 107, 109, 111
Rectus femoris 78, 80, 81, 91, 92
Recurrent back pain 3, 199
Reebok core board 112
Relaxin 206
Repetitions (Reps) 115, 143, 149, 151, 152, 153, 161, 162, 165, 166, 167, 170, 186, 188, 191, 192, 194, 195, 197
Resistance exercise continuum 150
Resistance training xii, 8, 9, 19, 76, 108, 112, 115, 130, 141, 147, 148, 149, 151, 152, 153, 154, 155, 156, 157, 158, 160, 161, 169
Resting heart rate 133, 134

Reverse fly 194, 195
Rheumatoid arthritis 115, 117
Rhomboids 93, 157, 179, 181, 190
Rotator cuff muscles 6, 19, 179
Rotators 22, 25, 59
Round shoulders 19

Sacral kyphosis 172
Sacroiliac joints 31, 63, 70, 75, 175, 204, 206
Sacrotuberous ligament 25
Sacrum 59, 60, 66, 70, 71, 172, 204
Sarcomere 6, 11, 46
Sarcoplasmic reticulum 10, 46
Satellite trigger points 51, 52, 54, 65, 69
Scheuermann's disease 178
Sciatic nerve 70, 86, 87
Sciatica xviii, 70, 86, 117, 177, 207
Scoliosis 51, 182, 183
Seated row 157, 190, 191
Self-myofascial release (SMR) 41, 42, 61, 74
Semimembranosus 78
Semitendinosus 78
Side plank 99, 100, 104, 105
Single-arm dumb-bell row 191
Sit-ups 26, 111, 122
Six-pack 20, 23, 27, 107, 109
Skeletal muscles 6, 43, 53
Sliding filament theory 10, 11
Slow-twitch (Type 1) fibres 6
Slumped posture 184
SMART principle 148
Smoking 16
Smooth muscles 5
Soleus 202
Spasm 26, 24, 44, 48, 185
Spinal mobilization exercises 33
Spinal twist 37

Spinalis 60
Spinous processes 21, 22, 23, 59, 60
Spondylolisthesis 4
Sports massage xi, xiii, 32, 35, 213, 215
Spray and stretch 73
Squats 96, 142, 156, 162
Stabilizer 6, 29, 94, 105, 106, 108, 111, 112, 154
Stabilizer muscles 6, 94, 105, 106, 111, 112
Static stretch 55, 77, 78, 148, 169
Sternocleidomastoid 181
Sternum 100, 190
Strength adaptation 155
Stretch reflex 53
Subacrominal space 19
Subacute back pain 3
Super slow 162
Superset 162, 164
Supination 200
Supraspinatus 19, 179
Sway back posture 184
Swiss ball 89, 95, 105, 106, 112, 114, 188
Synergist 25, 29, 30, 39, 41, 64, 69, 78, 84, 86, 98, 114, 154, 164, 175, 176, 185
Synergistic dominance 30, 64, 86, 175, 176, 185
Synovial 132, 148, 204

Tai chi 93
Tender points 55
Tens machines 35
Ten-second press test 56
Tensor fascia latae 25
Teres major 25
Theracane 58
Thermic effect of activity 118

Thermic effect of food 118, 119, 127
Thoracic kyphosis 172
Thoracolumbar fascia 23, 24, 25, 100
Tiberalis anterior 78
Tibia 48, 66, 78, 80, 84, 200, 202, 203
Transverse arch 201
Transverse processes 22, 23, 60, 61, 62, 80
Transversus abdominis 7, 23, 24, 31, 93, 100, 109, 111, 158, 160, 176, 187, 196
Transversus abdominis multifidus 7
Trapezius 49, 72, 93, 157, 179, 181, 190
Triceps 28, 29, 155, 157, 158, 164
Trigger point balls 58
Trigger points xiii, 4, 5, 30, 33, 34, 35, 38, 41, 42, 44, 45, 46, 47, 48, 49, 50, 51, 52, 53, 54, 55, 56, 57, 58, 59, 60, 61, 62, 63, 64, 65, 66, 67, 69, 70, 71, 72, 73, 74, 171, 172, 176, 181, 182, 185, 199, 205, 213, 215
Tri-set 161
Tropomyosin 10
Troponin 10
Twisting crunch 107, 189

Valsalva effect 156
Vastus lateralis 48, 91
Vastus medialis 48, 91

Warm-up 55, 131, 132, 148
Whey proteins 123
Xiphoid process 100

Yoga 93

ENDNOTES

1. Gordon Waddell, *The Back Pain Revolution*, 14.
2. Clark, Lucett, and Sutton, *NASM Corrective Exercise Training*, 1st ed. revised, chapter 2, 7.
3. Barry S. Levy, *Occupational and Environmental Health: Recognising and Preventing Disease and Injry*, 5th ed. (Philadelphia, 2006), 488-516.
4. C. Richardson, G. Jull, P. Hodges, and J. Hides, *Therapeutic Exercise for Spinal Segmental Stabilisation in Low Back Pain: Scientific Basis and Clinical Approach*, (Edinburgh, 1999).
5. Clark, Lucett, and Sutton, 25-29.
6. Travell and Simons, *Myofascial Pain & Dysfunction: The Trigger Point Manual* (1999).
7. Travell, J. and Simons, D. 1999. *Myofascial Pain & Dysfunction: The Trigger Point Manual.*
8. https://uk.images.search.yahoo.com/search/images;_ylt=A2KLn0WOIk1ay28A67hNBQx.?p=trigger+points&fr=yfp-t&imgl=fsuc&fr2=p%3As%2Cv%3Ai#id=38&iurl=https%3A%2F%2Fupload.wikimedia.org%2Fwikipedia%2Fcommons%2F7%2F72%2FTrigger_point_fibers.jpg&action=click
9. Travell, J. and Simons, D. 1999. *Myofascial Pain & Dysfunction: The Trigger Point Manual.* pp. 56-57.
10. Active IQ, *Level 4 Sports Massage Therapy Manual.*
11. Baechle Tr and Earle Rw. (2000), *Essentials of Strength Training and Conditioning*: 2nd Edition. Champaign, IL: Human Kinetics 8.
12. Travell, J. and Simons, D. 1999. *Myofascial Pain & Dysfunction: The Trigger Point Manual.*
13. Clark, Lucett, and Sutton, 64-65.
14. Bell, D.R., Padua, D.A. and Clark, M.A. 2008. "Muscle strength & flexibility characteristics of people displaying excessive medial knee displacement." *Arch Physical Med Rehabil.* 89: 1323-1328.

Printed in Great Britain
by Amazon